EMPOWERED MOTHERHOOD

NURTURING WELLNESS THROUGH PREGNANCY & BEYOND

CLAUDIA DUMOND

MINIMONDO

Copyright © 2024 Empowered Motherhood: Nurturing Wellness Through Pregnancy and Beyond by Claudia Dumond

All rights reserved. No part of this publication may be reproduced, distributed, or transmitted in any form or by any means, including photocopying, recording, or other electronic or mechanical methods, without the prior written permission of the publisher, except in the case of brief quotations embodied in critical reviews and certain other non-commercial uses permitted by copyright law.

This book is a work of nonfiction. The author has made every effort to ensure the accuracy of the information herein. However, the author and publisher assume no responsibility for errors, omissions, or damages caused by the use of the information contained herein.

ISBN: 9798341189195
Cover design: Claudia Dumond (w/ Canva)
Interior design: Claudia Dumond (w/ Canva)
Image Credits: www.unsplash.com (various photographers)
Independently Published By: Minimondo

THE CON- TENT

ABOUT US	5
INTRODUCTION	7
1. HEALTH AS A CORNERSTONE TO HAPPINESS	13
2. DISCOVERING YOUR TRUE SELF	35
3. DEBUNKING MOTHERHOOD MYTHS	51
4. MOTHERHOOD MINDSET SHIFTS	59
5. THE BODY - A MARVEL OF NATURE	75
6. STAY CONNECTED TO YOUR SOUL	91
7. CRAFTING YOUR UNIQUE WELLBEING TOOLKIT	101
8. WELLBEING TOOLKITS FOR EVERY MOOD	113
REFERENCES	121
ACKNOWLEDGEMENTS	123
ABOUT THE AUTHOR	125

ABOUT US

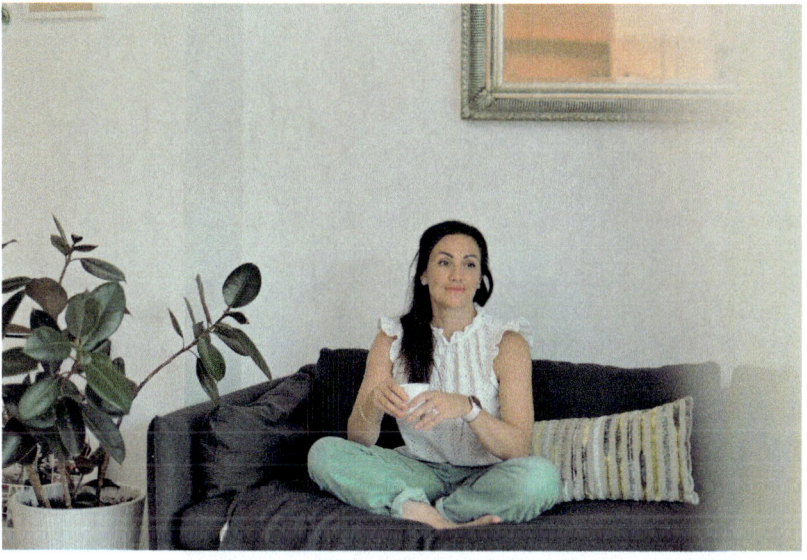

WWW.WEAREMINIMONDO.COM
WEAREMINIMGNDO@GMAIL.COM
@WEAREMINIMONDO

Welcome to *Minimondo*

The holistic wellness hub dedicated to enhancing your motherhood journey with joyful, healthy living. Our mission is to ensure you feel supported, vibrant and fulfilled every step of the way. With carefully crafted wellness services, from award-winning courses, content, coaching, and products, we empower pregnant women and beyond to design sustainable, healthy lifestyles that bring them joy and happiness, easing the transition to motherhood. We're the home of joyful wellbeing, empowering women to thrive on their journey through motherhood.

Claudia Dumond, our founder, brings over twenty years of experience in health and wellness to her role. She is passionately dedicated to nurturing sustainable wellness habits and empowering women to build holistic wellness toolkits to thrive during pregnancy and beyond. Please always consult your doctor before making significant lifestyle changes during pregnancy.

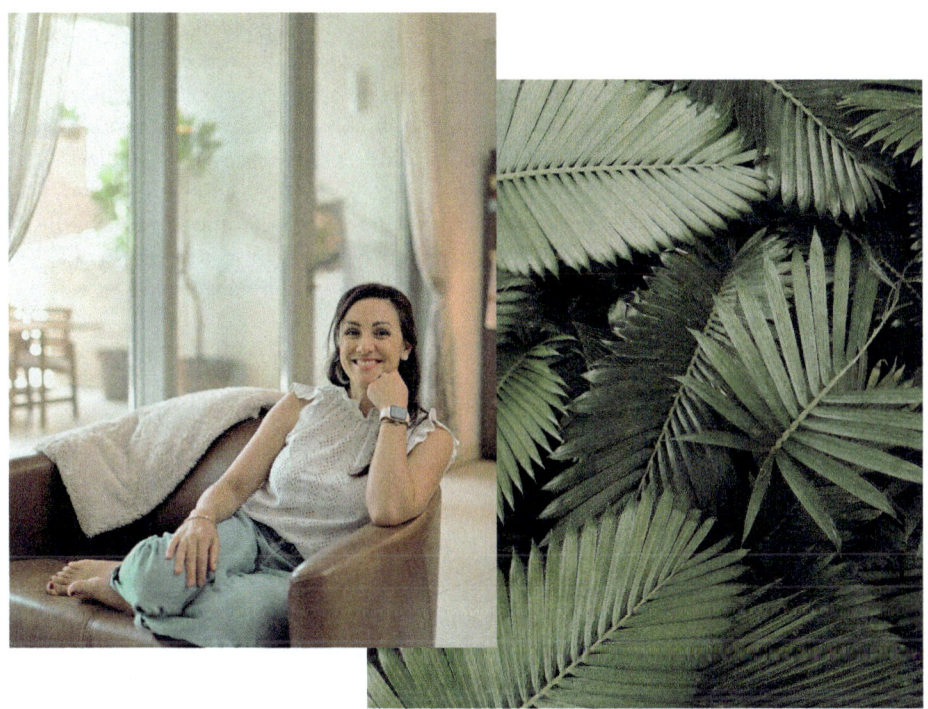

INTRODUCTION

Did you know that nearly two-thirds of women say they were unprepared for motherhood, including breastfeeding, mental health concerns, lack of sleep, and physical recovery from birth? And, whilst more than half of new mums created a plan for giving birth, only 11 percent made a plan for themselves and their recovery.[i] The reality is that shifting our focus towards our growing babies during pregnancy inevitably leads us to shift focus away from ourselves.

The truth is that motherhood is meant to be a transition. A transition to the new you, the becoming of a mother - It's called Matrescence.[ii] It's fair to say that motherhood is a time of profound transformation for women, both physically and emotionally. And whilst pregnancy is a special time to bond with your unborn child, what if you also used the next nine months as a unique opportunity to reconnect with yourself?

This book is designed to guide you through the transition to motherhood and prepare you with tools to ground you during this rollercoaster ride. Creating the tools to help build your confidence and curiosity is essential to ensuring a smoother journey to motherhood.

Pregnancy is the perfect time to focus on you. It is a time to understand your needs, wants, and hopes and to build healthy habits that will support you throughout your transition into motherhood. By prioritising your health, wellness, and wellbeing, and creating a unique wellbeing toolkit, we believe we can change the statistics around loneliness, identity loss, and other challenges new mothers face. Empowering yourself with this toolkit will help you thrive during pregnancy and provide a strong foundation for your journey through motherhood, ensuring you can handle any challenges with grace and confidence. Making conscious decisions and acting with intention will become your superpower through pregnancy and beyond.

I Wish I Were More Ready.

My first pregnancy was a breeze. Other than the odd hypochondriac, over-controlling first pregnancy jitters, it went by relatively unremarkable. My midwife appointments flew under the radar; I continued working in my fast-paced corporate job, read Lean In by Sheryl Sandberg (and did, with significant effect), and felt pretty good physically, too. I found a wonderful online pregnancy yoga class, walked halfway to work before waddling onto the tube, and did the same day after day. As I said, it was quite uneventful. I could say I was naively walking around in a reverie; one that I neither loathed nor loved, but a dream-like state, nonetheless.

It was time to wake up—and woke up I was.

It started during labour. That 48-hour labour that ended in a C-section, with too much anaesthetic administered, that I couldn't breathe appropriately whilst holding my baby for the first time. It took me three weeks to walk 100 metres outside with the baby as I recovered—very slowly. And so, it began. I was thrown a series of challenges that I can only say I was not ready for.

Above everything else was the challenge of sleep deprivation. For us, it was bad. Our son seemed to love a two-hour wake-up between one and three hours every single night, followed by a 4:30 am wake-up, for months. And he didn't really like a daytime nap much, either. The "sleep when the baby sleeps" just wasn't an option for me. I poured my time into figuring out how to fix the sleep problem. Then, finally, after ten months, we were cured with the help of a sleep consultant. The sun started to shine again, those black bags under our eyes began to retreat, and smiles returned to our faces. We emerged like moles after an extra-long hibernation. That was a challenging first year of motherhood. It turns out I wasn't ready.

And it didn't stop there, as the impending realisation that motherhood wasn't quite as wonderful, joyful, or fairy-tale-like set in, the absolute joy killer, Mr Comparison, came knocking at our door. We felt like we were in an eternal loop of purgatory, alive but not quite feeling like it.

It seemed that everyone else was skipping through fields of meadows. Their babies were sleeping through the night, chomping away on steaks, becoming musicians like Mozart, and living their best lives. We retreated even more. I wasn't ready.

Then came the invisible load that tends to fall on women's shoulders. I'm not blaming men here, by the way; I have an amazing husband who is very present. However, as he returned to work after a short but sweet paternity leave, I inevitably took on the house, home, and baby responsibilities. After my maternity leave, this did not change. I added full-time work to the list, plus nursery admin, drop-offs, pick-ups, and a second pregnancy, and so the weight started to pile onto my shoulders (and my previously flat stomach, too). I seriously wasn't ready.

With so much to do and what felt like so little time, I look back at those first few years as if I were a tornado whirling through life. And just like a tornado, I was a ball of nervous energy. I was changing form continually, both inside and out. My identity had changed, was changing, my body too, and I just didn't have an anchor point to bring me back down to earth. I was looking for a state of calm, of centredness, where I could trust my instincts as a new mother—a state where, despite everything changing, I could remain calm and handle it with grace and empathy. I wasn't ready, and because of it, I felt overwhelmed and out of control. I felt like I didn't know who I was anymore, what I liked—what I wanted. I was all consumed with my children and lost in the background. I was never alone, but I felt very lonely.

Why is This All Important?

The fact is, I wasn't alone after all. Loneliness in the first year of motherhood is more common than many of us realise. A recent survey has shown that 28% of new mothers experience loneliness after giving birth to their first child.[iii] The shift from being an independent individual to a mother can also lead to a significant loss of identity, with many women feeling as though they no longer know who they are outside of their role as a mother. This can be exacerbated by the pressures of modern motherhood, where the expectations to have it all and do it all are overwhelming.

Let's think about that for a second. A time that is meant to be the most beautiful bestowed to women, and they are dealing with struggles mentally, physically, and socially. So, what is going on exactly? Are women not supported enough? Is there too much information for women to get lost in that they don't trust their judgement enough? Are women mourning the loss of freedom after having children later in life? I don't think there is one thing to point to. What I do think is that women, whilst transitioning through one of the most significant changes of their lives, are just not ready. I, for one, was looking after myself through pregnancy, but I wasn't thinking about how to look after myself after becoming a mother.

When I was finally ready to come unstuck, I started reading lots of books, speaking to lots of other women, reading research papers, asking lots of questions, and then trying things that might help me feel more like myself again. I started step by step to build a wellbeing toolkit that I could turn to whenever life started to whirl back up again. This toolkit is filled with simple things. There are no magic creams for my cellulite and scars, no cold plunge pools in our home, no crazy expensive supplements, or silly diets to lose weight. My toolkit is filled with natural, sustainable, mindful, and simple wellness techniques across mind, body, and soul that bring me joy every single day. It is not one big thing, but lots of little things that help me make it through the day: my morning coffee, my breathing practices, my exercise routine (and my ability to easily flex it when needed). Most importantly, it is effective at grounding me when I get knocked off course and is unique to me and my lifestyle.

It's unbelievable, really, that the answers were always in front of me. I had the tools at my disposal, but I just didn't know I needed them in my most considerable time of need. I truly started to feel better and happier and to thrive again when I realised that a consistent, personalised, and holistic approach to health was the cornerstone to feeling good and tackling the transition to motherhood with grace and confidence. In fact, the importance of looking at health holistically—across mind, body, and soul—and building a wellbeing toolkit cannot be underestimated. And it is this that empowered me to find that calm and grounding that I was searching for.

What's a Wellbeing Toolkit?

Wellbeing is the quality of being healthy in body and mind to achieve a sense of joy in our lives, especially as an actively pursued goal. And a wellbeing toolkit is simply a collection of unique and personalised resources, actions, tools, and products that can be used to create a sense of wellbeing. If done properly, it becomes a way of life, a lifestyle. One that can give you an anchor point and a sense of centredness when life becomes chaotic and feels out of control. Having your own wellbeing toolkit will provide you with a sense of empowerment that leaves you feeling safe, knowing you have the tools to help yourself with whatever you're going through. Building your wellbeing toolkit takes time - It's a journey of exploration across mind, body, and soul. It's an opportunity to understand your wants, needs, passions, and interests, but it requires trial and error. Building your toolkit is the ultimate act of self-love and self-respect and is a beautiful, joyful journey to take and you have nine months to prepare to meet your newborn baby and the new you.

A holistic wellness toolkit will give you the confidence and courage to take on motherhood with calmness and grace—the chance to enjoy the process and the transition to the new you.

So, What's in It for You?

This book is for all the women out there who are preparing to step into motherhood. It's for those who want to create a solid foundation for their wellbeing to navigate this new chapter of their lives with confidence and resilience. By building your personalised wellbeing toolkit, you will have an anchor point to return to whenever you feel overwhelmed or lost. You will learn how to prioritise your physical and mental health, and you will understand why it's crucial for your happiness and the happiness of your family.

This book will break down wellbeing into six levers across mind, body, and soul so you can easily build a wellbeing toolkit with simple, manageable actions. Why do we call them levers? Because it emphasises that you are in control.

These levers are:

Mind Levers
Pause: Take moments to breathe, meditate, and be mindful.
Expand: Learn and grow through reading, education, creative, and exploration.

Body Levers
Move: Incorporate physical activity that suits your lifestyle and needs.
Food: Nourish your body with balanced, healthy meals.

Soul Levers
Space: Create a physical environment that supports your wellbeing.
Connect: Build and maintain supportive relationships.

In the following chapters, you will find practical advice, simple exercises, and tips to help you care for yourself across all these levers during pregnancy and beyond. You will discover ways to manage stress, maintain physical health, and nurture mental wellbeing. This is not about striving for perfection but finding your centre and creating a simple support system that works for you.

At the end of the book, you will have created a unique, personalised wellbeing toolkit that will empower you through your transition into motherhood and give you an anchor point to return to if or when motherhood throws you some curve balls. Because motherhood, despite all the cartoons we grow up with and their depiction of a fairytale, is hard.

Preparation and Prevention, not Treatment

Drawing on over twenty years in the health and wellness industry as a personal trainer, IIN-qualified health coach, award-winning course creator, consultant, and business owner, I want to help others to be ready.

Motherhood will throw different challenges to different women but one thing is for sure, we all deserve to enjoy motherhood from the get-go. I want women to enter motherhood with eyes wide open to help them build their own unique toolkit that might make their transition to motherhood more manageable and more joyful.

You have nine months to prepare for this transition. So, whilst you're choosing the baby car seat, the cot, the nursery colours, and the milk prep machine, remember to also focus on yourself. Give yourself the love you deserve across mind, body and soul throughout your pregnancy and beyond. Whilst you're getting ready for your new baby, make sure you're also preparing for the arrival of the new you.

Empowered motherhood is about preparation, not treatment. It's a call to action for women to pause and prepare themselves for the significant changes that come with motherhood. Investing in your wellbeing now will make the transition smoother and more joyful. This book is your guide to meeting your new self with grace, empathy, and confidence. Because you deserve to thrive, not just survive, in your journey through motherhood.

This book is your practical guide to creating a wellbeing toolkit that will help you thrive during motherhood. So, grab your pen and paper, and everywhere you see this symbol ✏️ is your moment to pause, reflect and take action. Now is the time to slow down, to get ready. Let's embark on this journey together, embracing each moment with mindfulness and intention. You'll learn to harness the power of your mind, body, and soul to create a balanced and fulfilling life for yourself and your baby.

Chapter One

HEALTH AS A CORNER-STONE TO HAPPINESS

Health encompasses physical, mental, and emotional wellbeing, serving as the foundation for a fulfilling life. Holistic health goes a step further by integrating these aspects, focusing on the whole person rather than just individual symptoms. At Minimondo, we focus on holistic health that touches the mind, body, and soul and we identify six wellbeing levers connected to these pillars. They are—Expand, Pause, Move, Food, Connect, and Space. These levers empower you to take control of your wellbeing, adjusting them as needed to suit your evolving lifestyle.

During pregnancy, understanding these levers will help you build a comprehensive toolkit, enabling you to create a balanced and fulfilling life for yourself and your baby. In this chapter, we delve into the wellbeing levers in depth and introduce you to some wellbeing principles that can help you navigate this transformative journey confidently and easily by recognising what brings you joy and fulfilment.

> "
> **WHEN IT COMES TO WHOLENESS, WE'RE NEVER QUITE AS CLOSE AS WE THINK, BUT WE'RE ALSO NEVER AS FAR AS WE FEAR.**

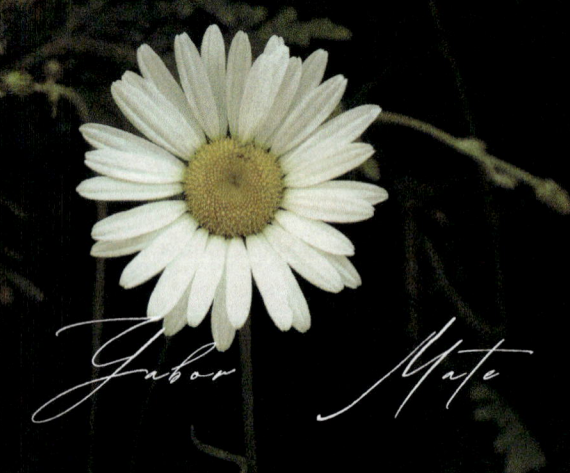

— *Gabor Maté*

The Transformative Power of *holistic health*

The connection between the mind, body, and soul is a fundamental concept that has gained increasing attention in modern research and holistic health practices. This triad represents the interdependence of our mental, physical, and spiritual wellbeing, suggesting that we achieve true health when all three are in harmony. Numerous studies have shown that mental health can directly impact physical health, with chronic stress, for instance, being linked to conditions such as heart disease, weakened immune function, and digestive issues. Conversely, physical activity has been proven to boost mental health by reducing symptoms of anxiety and depression. Spiritual wellbeing, often nurtured through practices like meditation or mindfulness, has also been shown to enhance both mental clarity and physical resilience.

As an expectant mother, you embark on a remarkable journey that involves nurturing a new life and yourself. Pregnancy presents a unique opportunity to delve into holistic wellbeing, understanding the intricate facets that compose your health and contribute to your happiness. Prioritising holistic health during pregnancy sets the stage for a fulfilling journey into motherhood and beyond. By embracing nourishing foods, engaging in gentle physical activity, cultivating mindfulness and self-awareness, nurturing meaningful connections, and aligning with your core values and purpose, you can establish a robust foundation for lasting happiness and wellbeing.

As we embark on this journey together, let's remember that happiness is not merely a destination but a way of being—a state cultivated through conscious choices and holistic practices. I invite you to explore the principles of holistic health and commit to your wellness journey. Let's start with visiting intrinsic and extrinsic wellbeing.

Intrinsic Vs. Extrinsic
wellbeing

Intrinsic: Intrinsic wellbeing refers to a deep, internal sense of satisfaction and contentment that arises from within, driven by personal values, self-acceptance, and a sense of purpose. It's about finding joy in the process of living and engaging in activities that resonate with your true self. As you transition into motherhood, this type of wellbeing becomes incredibly important. It's about staying connected to your sense of self, practicing self-acceptance as your body and life change, and finding joy in the small moments. Cultivating intrinsic wellbeing involves listening to your intuition, engaging in activities that align with your true self, and embracing the journey rather than focusing solely on the destination. This inner contentment is crucial during pregnancy and early motherhood, as it helps you navigate challenges with resilience and grace, creating a strong foundation for both you and your child. By nurturing your intrinsic wellbeing, you empower yourself to face the uncertainties of motherhood with confidence and calm, knowing that your sense of happiness and purpose comes from within.

Extrinsic: Extrinsic wellbeing involves recognising how the environment—including the spaces, places, and people we surround ourselves with—can significantly impact our mental and physical health. As your body and life undergo profound changes, the spaces you inhabit, the people you interact with, and even the sensory elements in your environment—like lighting, scents, and sounds—can impact your overall wellbeing. Creating a nurturing, supportive environment becomes essential; this could mean decluttering your living space to reduce stress or surrounding yourself with a strong support system. The relationships you maintain and the community you build play a pivotal role in your extrinsic wellbeing, offering emotional support and practical help when needed. By consciously designing an environment that promotes relaxation, comfort, and positivity, you can enhance your well-being and better support your transition into motherhood. This balanced approach ensures that both your inner and outer worlds are aligned to foster a healthy, fulfilling experience during pregnancy and beyond.

When we have strength internally, we can succeed at anything. Combine this with the right things around us and a fulfilling experience during pregnancy and beyond is inevitable.

Wellbeing *levers*

Wellbeing levers are integral components that contribute to overall health and happiness. Whilst each lever can be looked at individually, they are deeply interconnected. In fact, the true essence of wellbeing emerges from understanding how these elements interact and support one another—that optimising one area often enhances others, creating a harmonious and holistic approach to wellbeing.

The Mind (Pause and Expand Levers)

The mind is deeply affected during pregnancy and the postnatal period, with significant hormonal shifts influencing mental and emotional health. For example, increased levels of progesterone and oestrogen can lead to heightened emotions, mood swings, and even anxiety or depression. Research indicates that up to one in five women will experience mental health issues during pregnancy or in the first year after birth.[iv] Cognitive changes, often referred to as "baby brain," can also occur, with many women reporting forgetfulness or difficulty concentrating. However, with awareness and the proper support, these challenges can be managed, allowing mothers to maintain a strong, positive mindset as they navigate their new role.

To nurture your mind, we focus on:

- **Pause Lever:** Bringing our minds back to the present and finding ways to slow down and be more present (e.g. practising mindfulness, meditation, or slowing down).
- **Expand Lever:** Encouraging curiosity to nourish our minds in the right way to support continuous growth, enabling us to tap back into our spark (e.g. continuous learning, finance, career, hobbies, and expression).

The Body (Food and Move Levers)

Physically, the body undergoes dramatic changes during pregnancy and childbirth. The surge of relaxin, a hormone that loosens ligaments and joints, prepares the body for birth but can also lead to aches and pains, particularly in the pelvis and lower back. After birth, women face the challenge of recovering from childbirth, which may include healing from tears, caesarean sections, or other physical traumas. The body also adjusts to the demands of breastfeeding, which can impact sleep, energy levels, and physical comfort. Understanding these changes and nurturing the body through proper nutrition, exercise, and rest is essential to regaining strength and vitality.

To nurture your body, we focus on:

- **Food Lever:** Being in tune with our body and focusing on the right ingredients to achieve a healthy mind and body through food (e.g. types of food, amount of water, and home cooking).
- **Move Lever:** Being in tune with our body and focusing on the right types of movement to achieve optimal health (e.g. being active, type of exercise, rest and sleep).

The Soul (Connect and Space Levers)

The soul, representing the more profound, spiritual aspect of a woman's wellbeing, is often transformed as she steps into motherhood. This transition can bring a deep sense of purpose and fulfilment, but it can also challenge a woman's sense of identity and connection to herself. The loss of personal time, the intensity of caring for a newborn, and the societal pressures to be the perfect mother can lead to feelings of isolation or loss of self. However, by nurturing the soul—through practices like mindfulness, connection with others, and self-reflection—women can find a new sense of self that is enriched by their journey into motherhood.

Here, we explore:

- **Connect Lever:** Focusing on our innate need to connect with ourselves and others. Be it personal, social, or through giving back (e.g. joy with others and deep connection with oneself and others)
- **Space Lever**: Making sure that the space around us works hard to build up our energy supply in the right way (e.g. space design (home/office) and being surrounded by nature).

Getting started
with wellbeing

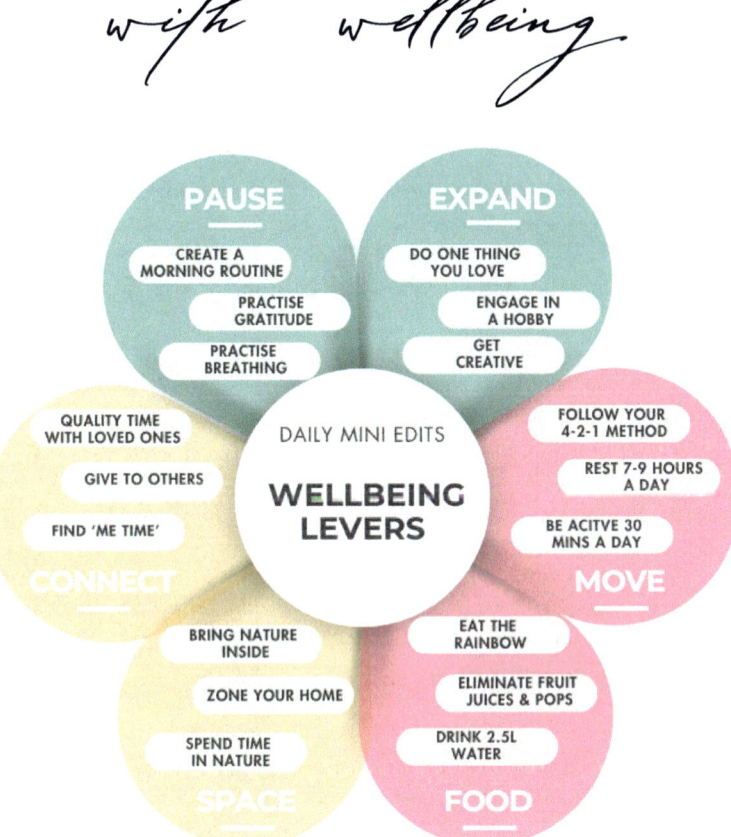

Embracing Curiosity: A Pathway to Nurturing Wellbeing During Pregnancy

During pregnancy, it's vital to embrace a sense of curiosity, examine areas of your life that could benefit from improvement, and discover the healthy habits that bring you joy. This is a time to fearlessly explore, to try new things, and to cultivate a growth mindset. Motherhood demands adaptability and positivity, and the nine months of pregnancy are an ideal opportunity to identify what truly lights you up. The transition to motherhood can feel less overwhelming by fostering curiosity and flexibility now. Starting with small, sustainable, healthy habits is a great way to lay a solid foundation for this journey. It's not just about daily adjustments; it's about preparing mentally and emotionally for the beautiful journey ahead. The diagram above shows some small edits you can start thinking about adopting in your daily life.

Principles
of wellbeing

At Minimondo, we believe that true wellbeing is grounded in four guiding principles: simplicity, natural choices, sustainability, and joy. Simplicity encourages us to start small, focusing on manageable changes that can have a significant impact over time. It's about making "mini edits" to our lives, which can lead to lasting improvements.

The natural principle emphasises the importance of choosing foods, products, and environments as close to nature as possible—offering holistic benefits that artificial alternatives simply can't match.

Sustainability ensures that the habits we adopt are not just fleeting trends but practices we can maintain for the long haul, avoiding the pitfalls of short-lived fads.

Focusing on simplicity is also key. The clue is in the name, why complicate wellbeing when you can choose simple and easy habits that can bring lots of joy? This is not about the big elaborate holiday every year (although there is a place for that too). This is about finding small and easy things that help to optimise your health and are super easy to stick to.

Finally, and most importantly, we prioritise joy. Building healthy habits that bring us genuine happiness is vital to ensuring that we stick with them. When we find pleasure in the habits that support our wellbeing, we're much more likely to make them a lasting part of our lives. By being mindful and intentional about embracing these four principles, you can create a powerful foundation for lasting, positive change.

THE POWER OF SIMPLICITY

The principle of simplicity in wellbeing is about embracing the power of small, manageable changes that can make a significant impact over time. When we approach wellbeing with simplicity in mind, it becomes less overwhelming and more accessible, allowing us to integrate healthy habits into our lives more easily. For expectant mothers and new mums, simplicity in healthy habits can make the difference between feeling overwhelmed and empowered to nurture their wellbeing.

At Minimondo, we focus on mini edits.

What's a mini edit? It's a way of thinking.

The concept of mini edits is about making small yet meaningful changes to our daily routines to foster a positive journey towards wellbeing. These edits aren't overwhelming; they're manageable tweaks you can consistently integrate into your life. Whether adding a few minutes of mindfulness each day or making healthier food choices, mini edits help us continually improve and adjust as we navigate pregnancy and motherhood. By embracing these small changes, we create a sustainable path to wellbeing that evolves with us.

For the mind, simplicity can begin with just a minute of mindfulness or reflection each day. For instance, journaling your thoughts a minute before bed can help clear your mind and promote better sleep. This small practice can be a powerful tool for mental clarity and emotional balance, as it creates a dedicated space to process your day and set intentions for tomorrow.

In terms of the body, starting with simple, short exercises can build a sustainable routine. For example, a minute of sit-ups before your morning shower may not seem like much, but it's a small step towards creating physical strength and establishing a habit of daily movement. Over time, these minutes can add up, making exercise a regular part of your routine without feeling like a burden.

For the soul, simplicity might mean incorporating brief moments of joy and self-affirmation into your day. Before getting out of bed, spend a minute focusing on your breathing and reciting affirmations that uplift and centre you.

This small act can set a positive tone for the day ahead, nurturing your inner self and reinforcing a sense of purpose and peace.

This act of starting the day with positive statements was such a powerful tool for me. Before I even opened my eyes, I would remind myself of all the love I have for my family and all the positive things in my life, and I reminded myself to tackle the day with positivity and love. These are some of the statements I would recite to set me up for the day ahead:

- Today, I choose to find joy in the little moments, to laugh often, and to let go of what I cannot control.
- I will approach every task with a calm heart and a clear mind.
- Today, I will embrace the journey of motherhood with patience and love, knowing that each challenge is an opportunity to grow.
- I will nurture myself as much as I nurture my child, recognising that my wellbeing is essential to being the best mother I can be.
- Today, I will lead with kindness—towards my child, my partner, and myself—creating a home filled with warmth and understanding.

"GETTING HEALTHY IS JUST FOR THE WEALTHY"

- BREATHWORK $0
- NATURE $0
- MEDITATION $0
- GRATITUDE $0
- GROUNDING $0
- SUNSHINE $0
- WALKING $0
- COMMUNITY $0
- YOGA $0
- PRIORITIZING SLEEP $0
- SPIRITUAL PRACTICE $0
- INTERMITTENT FASTING $0
- NOT COMPLAINING $0
- TURNING WIFI OFF AT NIGHT $0
- PICKING UP HEAVY THINGS $0
- NOT DRINKING ALCOHOL $0
- A "WHY" BIGGER THAN EXCUSES $0
- WALKING AWAY FROM YOUR PHONE $0
- STOP EATING OUT SO MUCH $0
- NOT BUYING FOODS THAT DON'T LOVE YOU BACK $0

DR. WILL COLE

THE POWER OF NATURAL

From a walk in the park or simply sitting in a garden, to using natural products to minimise exposure to harmful chemicals, choosing natural practises and products can reduce stress and elevate mood. In fact, research consistently shows that spending time in nature reduces stress, anxiety, and depression. One revealed that just twenty minutes in a park can reduce cortisol levels by nearly 20 percent.[v] What's more is that these natural practices are often free, making them easily accessible and sustainable. By consciously choosing natural options, we can make a profound impact on our wellbeing, creating a healthier and more balanced life.

For the mind, using natural scents like lavender or chamomile in aromatherapy can promote relaxation and improve sleep quality, supporting mental clarity and reducing stress. In fact, the sense of smell is a powerful tool for creating and reinforcing associations, especially during transformative periods like pregnancy and motherhood. The phenomenon is rooted in how our brain processes scents, primarily through the olfactory system, which is closely linked to the limbic system—the part of the brain responsible for emotions and memory.

Lavender, for example, is well-known and researched for its calming properties. It has been shown to reduce anxiety, improve sleep quality, and lower stress levels. During pregnancy, you can start building a positive association with lavender by carrying a small bottle of essential oil with you. Whenever you feel calm, take a moment to inhale the scent for about a minute. Repeating this practice throughout your pregnancy can create a strong link between the scent of lavender and a sense of calm. Then, when you face challenges or stress as a new mother, the simple act of smelling lavender can help your nervous system return to a place of calm because you've established this association.

Other essential oils that offer similar benefits include chamomile, known for its gentle calming effects, and borgamot, which can help lift your mood and reduce feelings of anxiety. As with any essential oil, ensuring that the one you choose is safe for use during pregnancy is important. This practice of using natural scents to foster calmness and positivity can be a valuable addition to your wellbeing toolkit as you navigate the journey into motherhood.

For the body, embracing natural foods, such as fresh fruits and vegetables, whole grains, and lean proteins, provides essential nutrients that support energy levels, digestion, and overall health. For example, leafy greens like spinach and kale are rich in vitamins and antioxidants that help reduce inflammation and boost the immune system.

When it comes to the soul, connecting with nature or bringing natural elements into our homes—like plants or natural light—has been shown to foster feelings of calm and improve mood. Even something as simple as a few minutes in a garden or incorporating houseplants into your living space can create a more serene environment.

THE POWER OF SUSTAINABLE

When we talk about sustainable choices in the context of wellbeing, we're referring to the idea of making realistic and lasting changes that seamlessly fit into our lives. Unlike drastic overhauls or extreme measures that might be short-lived, sustainable practices focus on gradual adjustments that we can maintain over the long term. The goal is to find a balance that supports continuous improvement without overwhelming us, ensuring that our new habits can become an integral part of our everyday routines. This requires being honest with yourself about what you can realistically maintain. If a new habit is expensive, you might only stick to it briefly before financial concerns lead you to stop.

Similarly, it might become exhausting over time if it demands getting up an hour earlier than usual to go to the gym every day. When introducing healthy habits, consider how likely they are to be sustainable and long-lasting. Aim for habits that fit seamlessly into your lifestyle, ensuring they become enduring practices rather than fleeting changes. Sustainable habits are crucial to lasting positive lifestyle changes supporting your health and wellbeing.

For the mind, rather than committing to lengthy meditation sessions right away, start with just five minutes a day and gradually extend your practice as it becomes more comfortable. Alternatively, integrate mindfulness into your existing routines, such as practising brief breathing exercises whilst commuting or in the shower.

For physical wellbeing, focus on making incremental dietary and fitness changes that are practical and long-lasting. Instead of jumping into extreme diets or expensive fitness regimes, address one aspect of your diet, such as reducing sugary drinks or processed foods. A quick tip is to toss all the processed foods from your cupboards and start replacing them with healthier options. Similarly, establish a workout routine that fits your current lifestyle and budget, such as incorporating short, daily exercise sessions or exploring free online resources. These small, consistent adjustments can lead to sustainable improvements without requiring drastic changes or significant financial commitments.

I've tried many times over to get myself up an hour earlier each day because I want to fit a workout in before the boys go to school, but my body just keeps resisting it. I just cannot commit to it long-term, and boy, have I tried. So, for now, I'm accepting that it just isn't for me and finding ways to fit in workouts that don't require me to wake up before the sun comes up.

Sustaining emotional and spiritual wellbeing involves engaging in small yet meaningful activities that align with your values and bring joy. This might include dedicating a few minutes to personal reflection or journaling regularly, participating in small acts of kindness, or nurturing connections with your community. Making these practices a regular part of your routine creates a sense of fulfilment and belonging that supports long-term emotional and spiritual health.

THE POWER OF JOY

Joy is perhaps the most essential principle of wellbeing. It is a profound sense of happiness and contentment that arises from within. Unfortunately, wellbeing practices sometimes get a bad rap for being restrictive or burdensome. The true essence of a wellbeing toolkit is understanding and embracing what genuinely brings you happiness. This personal exploration is vital to developing habits that not only benefit your health but also enrich your life. If a rigorous gym session feels more like a chore than a pleasure, consider alternatives like a refreshing walk or a run in the park. The joy you find in your wellbeing practices will naturally make you more inclined to stick with them.

When it comes to mental wellbeing, focus on activities that ignite your passion and creativity. Reflect on what used to bring you joy in your younger years—whether it was painting, writing, or playing a musical instrument. Rediscovering these interests can rekindle a sense of fulfilment and motivation. Consider keeping a mood diary as you explore new activities to track which ones lift your spirits the most. For instance, if singing in a choir or spending time in nature brings you joy, consider how you can continue these activities even after becoming a mother. Plan by arranging support systems—perhaps finding a caregiver for your baby whilst you attend your favourite yoga class or scheduling weekly nature outings, whatever the weather.

For physical wellbeing, prioritise joyful movement over rigorous exercise routines that may not suit you. Instead of forcing yourself into an intense gym programme, find forms of exercise that you look forward to, such as dancing, swimming, or hiking in nature. The goal is to integrate movement into your life in a way that feels enjoyable rather than obligatory. Experiment with different activities and observe which ones make you feel happy and invigorated. This approach ensures that staying active becomes a pleasurable part of your routine rather than a burdensome task.

As a personal trainer, I never expected that becoming a mother would affect my love of fitness or being active, but of all the changes that happened to me, this was the most significant change. I didn't plan for how to stay active once becoming a mother; I didn't anticipate the guilt that would set in when leaving my children to go to the gym instead of spending time with them. In the end, this part of getting back on track has been the most challenging part of my life. Mainly because I was expecting to continue exercising as I used to before having a baby—going to the gym five times a week—and when I could not continue this way, due to both time and financial pressures,

I got stuck in a rut. Over time, and with lots of trial and testing, I have found a wonderful routine that works for the children and me. I have sectioned off a corner of the house so I can do Pilates a few times a week using an app I love (Alo Moves). I go for walks and runs outside (weather permitting) and I try to stretch as much as possible to keep nimble (this strangely happens under a nice hot shower, of all places). But hey, that's what a unique wellbeing toolkit looks like; it fits like a glove into my lifestyle!

Nurturing your soul involves surrounding yourself with people, places, and activities that bring genuine happiness. As you prepare for your baby's arrival, create spaces and routines that nurture your soul and provide moments of respite and joy. These considerations enhance your wellbeing and support your transition into motherhood. Reflect on the social connections, environments, and experiences that resonate with you deeply.

Designing a personal retreat space in your home can provide a much-needed sanctuary where you can find solace and joy amidst the demands of new motherhood. Consider carving out a small nook or corner dedicated to activities that bring you happiness. This might be a cosy reading corner with your favourite books and a comfortable chair, a space where you can play uplifting music, or a spot where you can light a candle that evokes a sense of calm and joy. A designated area for relaxation and self-care can offer a peaceful retreat when you need a break and help you maintain a sense of personal wellbeing.

Also, consider building a robust support network to help you navigate this new chapter's challenges and joys. Start by identifying and nurturing relationships with family members, friends, and community resources you can rely on and be clear about the role you would like them to play in your and your child's life. Reflect on the people, places, and activities that bring you genuine joy, and make time for them even after your baby arrives. This could involve maintaining connections with close friends or simply finding moments for solitude and relaxation. By continuing to nurture these aspects of your life, you ensure your happiness and wellbeing remain a priority.

Micro-Moments
of joy

The other thing to think about when it comes to joy is focusing on micro-moments of joy—those small, everyday experiences that make you smile and lift your spirit. Micro moments of joy are the small, often fleeting instances of happiness or contentment that occur throughout our day. These moments can range from the warmth of a sunny morning, a smile from a stranger, or a brief but meaningful conversation with a friend. They are subtle yet powerful, often overlooked in the hustle of daily life. Try to become aware of these small moments as these are the ones that become the most important in the routine of motherhood.

If you prioritise activities that bring you genuine joy, they will become lasting habits rather than fleeting efforts. By finding joy in the practices across the six levers of wellbeing that genuinely light you up, you're much more likely to stick to a healthy lifestyle and fall in love with the journey. Joyful practices and micro-moments of joy create a positive and sustainable approach to wellbeing, making your healthy lifestyle a source of happiness and fulfilment.

> **OUR MOST PRECIOUS COMMODITY THESE DAYS IS TIME, SO A SUPPER TOGETHER, OR A LONG PHONE CALL MIGHT HAVE INFINITELY MORE VALUE THAN A RANDOM ACQUISITION.**

Michelle Ogundehin

Check in on
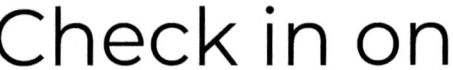

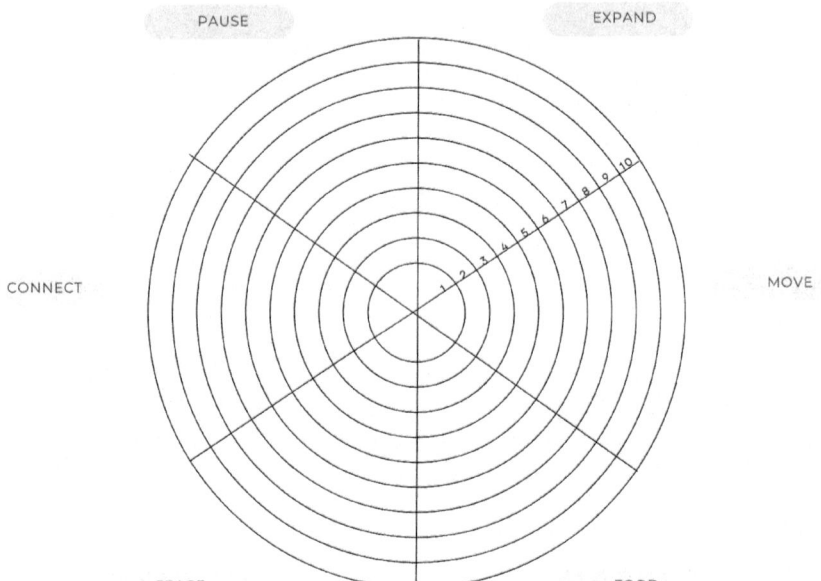

Pause and reflect on your current lifestyle across the six wellbeing levers, considering what enables you to feel healthy, confident and joyful. Assess your healthy habits within each lever on a scale of 1 to 10 (10 = doing great, 1 = could do better), acknowledging what's already working well for you and what is driving your actions.

This introspection forms the foundation for enhancing your wellbeing and preparing for motherhood. Let's honour your strengths and identify areas for growth as we journey together.

What's Working Well Today and Why?

Use some of these prompts to help you think about your daily habits today and to start to get under the skin of whether you are creating a lifestyle that is both sustainable and joyful once your baby arrives:

- How do I currently manage stress? Are these methods effective, or do I need to explore new strategies?
- Am I engaging in activities that stimulate my personal development? What are my current learning or growth goals?
- Is my current exercise routine enjoyable and sustainable? Am I consistent with my physical activity, and does it align with my fitness goals?
- Am I satisfied with my diet? Are there areas where I could improve?
- Do I feel emotionally fulfilled and content? Are there aspects of my life where I lack joy or satisfaction?
- Am I nurturing meaningful relationships with friends and family? Do I feel supported and understood by those around me?
- How actively am I building and nurturing my support network? Are there opportunities to connect with others who share my interests or values?
- Do I have a reliable support network in place? Are there specific areas where I need more support or assistance?
- Are my daily activities and choices aligned with my core values and beliefs? How well am I honouring what is important to me?

A Quick Recap

In this chapter, we focused on health as the foundation of happiness, supported by a balanced approach across mind, body, and soul. The six key levers—pause, expand, move, food, connect, and space—help create a well-rounded sense of wellbeing. By focusing on sustainability, joy, simplicity, and natural choices, wellbeing can become a lifestyle, not just a temporary fad—allowing us to grow and find happiness in everyday life.

Key Points:

- **The connection between mind, body, and soul:** Health is built on the connection between mind, body, and soul, creating a holistic sense of wellbeing.
- **Levers of wellbeing allow us to be in control:** The six key levers—pause, expand, move, food, connect, and space—give us agency in creating a healthy lifestyle that is within our control.
- **Focus on four wellbeing principles:** When introducing new healthy habits, think about the four principles of wellbeing—Sustainable, Natural, Simple, Joyful.
- **Micro moments of joy:** Focusing on the little things that bring a smile to your face every single day will create a strong grounding for committing to healthy habits.
- **Embrace curiosity:** Be curious as you journey through creating your wellbeing toolkit. There is no right answer. Try some things, become aware of what is working (and what isn't) and switch it up until you find something that's going to stick.

Chapter Two

DISCOVER-ING YOUR TRUE SELF

Change is an intrinsic part of becoming a mother. As you transition into this new role, you may encounter a whirlwind of emotional, physical, and practical changes that redefine your routines and perspectives. Embracing this transformation means acknowledging and accepting the evolving nature of your life, from adjusting to new responsibilities and routines to nurturing a deep bond with your baby. Whilst change can be challenging, it also presents an opportunity for growth and self-discovery. By approaching this journey with flexibility and an open heart, you can navigate the changes with resilience, finding new strengths and joys in the beautiful evolution of motherhood.

The journey to creating your unique wellbeing toolkit begins with the desire to truly understand yourself. It starts with recognising your wants and needs and deeply examining your belief system. By first aligning your thoughts with the person you aspire to become, you lay the foundation for meaningful change. Pregnancy and early motherhood bring a whirlwind of emotions, often driven by fluctuating hormones. Still, once you cultivate the mindset of the person you want to be, you can begin to engage in actions that reflect this new identity. As you consistently practice these aligned behaviours, positive feelings and lasting satisfaction will naturally follow.

"

THE MOMENT A CHILD IS BORN, THE MOTHER IS ALSO BORN.

Osho

Your unique *wellbeing Toolkit*

Your wellbeing toolkit will be a collection of strategies, resources, and practices to help you improve and maintain your overall wellbeing through mind, body, and soul. Just as every mother and every child is wonderfully unique, your wellbeing toolkit will be bespoke to you. Whether your toolkit is filled with simple, small habits or elaborate self-care rituals, the key is that it reflects what genuinely helps you feel centred, supported, and energised.

Motherhood is a transformative experience, a beautiful yet unpredictable rollercoaster of emotions. There will be days of unparalleled joy and moments of overwhelming challenge. By building your wellbeing toolkit now, you're laying the groundwork for a more balanced and fulfilling motherhood journey. This toolkit will be your anchor, providing stability and comfort when the waves of life get choppy. In this chapter, we will introduce you to a new way of thinking, one that will underpin how you create and apply your unique wellbeing toolkit and equipping you with the tools to thrive as you embrace the incredible adventure of motherhood.

Think. Do. *Feel.*

The Think-Do-Feel Model underscores that transformation starts from within. Creating a harmonious path from thought to action to emotion. Whilst you can't control every feeling, you can effectively develop strategies to manage these emotional tides. The Think-Do-Feel Model offers a comprehensive approach to help you understand and navigate your emotions by integrating cognitive (think), behavioural (do), and emotional (feel) strategies. This model empowers you to truly stick to healthy habits that will support you through the transition into motherhood.

THINK: The Foundation of Transformation

Transformation begins in the "Think" phase, rooted in cognitive strategies that shape our mindset and behaviour. Your wellbeing toolkit starts here. It's crucial to first clarify the type of lifestyle you aspire to, understand who you are as a person, and clarify your core values. This mental clarity acts as your North Star, guiding every decision and action.

Research shows that setting clear, values-based goals and having a strong sense of identity significantly enhances motivation and commitment. In fact, people who set goals aligned with their personal values are more likely to persist in their efforts and achieve long-term success.[vi] By defining your desired lifestyle and self-concept, you create a solid foundation for making choices that resonate with your authentic self, ensuring that your actions are sustainable and deeply fulfilling.

Since becoming a mother, I have spent a significant amount of time getting back to my values and sense of self. I have defined these values as Freedom, Loyalty, Peace, Adventure, and Health. These five simple words have formed the foundation for how I choose to live my life. My values have significantly influenced my actions, from my decisions around work and finances to how I want to parent my children. For example, I have always loved travelling as it fills me with a sense of adventure and curiosity that I struggle to find in my everyday life, and this has led to my husband and me choosing to live for a few years outside of our home town—even though it was a difficult and frightening decision, this is so directly aligned with my sense of self that we have never looked back no matter how hard it has been to leave family behind.

DO: Taking Aligned Action.

The "Do" phase focuses on implementing actions that align with your values, sense of self, and belief system. This phase is about translating your cognitive clarity into tangible, purposeful steps that resonate with who you are and want to become. By connecting your actions to the six wellbeing levers, you create a clear framework for decision-making. This approach not only helps you prioritise actions that are most meaningful to you but also provides a simple checkpoint for evaluating where to invest your time and energy. As you navigate the demands of motherhood and face challenges like limited time or feelings of mum guilt, having a clear alignment between your values and actions allows you to use your time wisely and mitigate any associated guilt. Research supports that goal alignment with personal values enhances motivation and reduces stress, leading to more effective and satisfying outcomes.[vii] Focusing on actions that truly matter to you ensures that every step you take is purposeful and in harmony with your overall sense of self and wellbeing.

FEEL: The Power of Emotions in Sustaining Change

The "Feel" aspect delves into the emotional responses that arise from our actions and their role in reinforcing healthy habits. More often than not, we allow our actions to be dictated by how we feel. Maybe we laze in front of the TV in the evening instead of preparing a healthy lunch for the next day or we reach for the sugary snack in the afternoon when we are having a lull. In reality, we must use our actions to help impact our emotions more.

By becoming aware of how specific activities impact our emotions—such as experiencing joy and strength from daily walks in nature—we can harness these positive feelings to reinforce our identity and motivation. Positive emotions act as powerful motivators, reinforcing the habits that contribute to our desired sense of self. For example, research highlights that engaging in activities that evoke pleasure and satisfaction not only enhances our emotional wellbeing but also increases the likelihood of maintaining those behaviours over time.[viii] By recognising and embracing the feelings associated with your actions, you create a feedback loop where positive emotions strengthen your commitment to healthy habits, making it easier to sustain the changes that align with who you are and who you aspire to become. This mindful approach to emotions ensures that your wellbeing journey is not only effective but also deeply meaningful.

THINK
BE CLEAR ON
YOUR VALUES &
IDENTITY

EVIDENCE   MOTIVATION

**FEELINGS
FOLLOW
ACTION**

@weareminimondo

FEEL
FEEL YOUR HAPPY
HORMONE KICK IN
AND THE CHANGE
IN EMOTIONS

DO
TAKE SMALL
HEALTHY ACTIONS
ALIGNED TO YOUR
VALUES

DOPAMINE

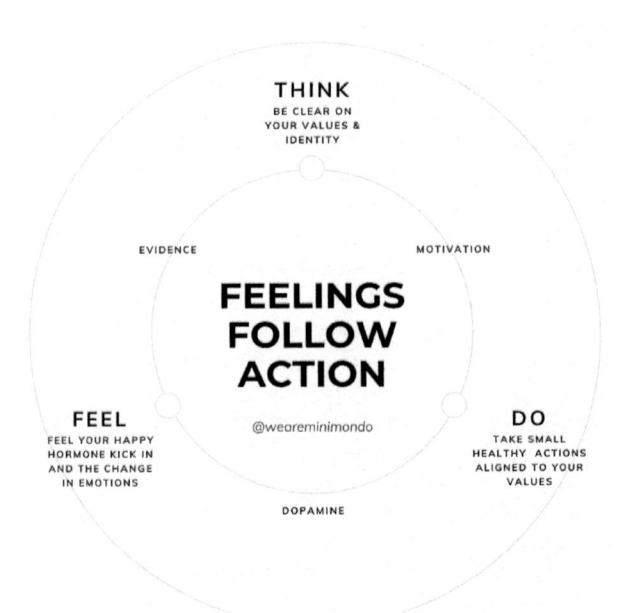

FEELINGS FOLLOW ACTION

The emotional journey of motherhood is as varied and complex as the ocean's tides. Embrace the changing tides and know you are not alone in feeling this way. Your feelings are a testament to the profound and beautiful experience of becoming a mother. But, sometimes, letting our feelings dictate our actions and waiting for motivation to strike becomes a harder journey to wellbeing. This proactive method helps ensure consistency, allowing you to enjoy the rewards of a healthier, happier lifestyle. And by identifying simple, natural, sustainable and joyful actions, you can more effectively incorporate them into your daily routine and create a joyful approach to wellbeing.

When I first became a mother, I now realise that I relied too heavily on my fluctuating feelings to dictate how my day would unfold. Most of the time, I felt utterly exhausted, both physically and emotionally. This led me to simply survive each day rather than truly live it. Looking back, I see that I could have incorporated simple practices from the start that aligned with my sense of self, which might have prevented me from losing myself so much in the process. I would have established a powerful internal motivation system if I had done this. I could have asked for help more often, allowing me to take short walks alone to clear my mind. I could have set aside an hour each week to engage in something I loved. I could have taken ten minutes a day to stretch or lift some weights which could have energised me and brought me joy, fostering a more balanced and fulfilling experience of motherhood. That's the power of the Think-Do-Feel Model and the importance of putting it into practise during pregnancy so that you continue to incorporate healthy habits and focus on some of the things that bring you the most joy as you enter into motherhood.

It starts with
your values

A profound journey of self-discovery is at the heart of building lasting, positive habits. Before diving into the realm of new routines and changes, it's essential first to explore and define your core values. Understanding your authentic identity provides a solid foundation for creating habits that truly resonate with who you are.

In this process, we'll embark on activities designed to help you uncover and articulate the values that are most meaningful to you. By focusing on just a few defining words, you can rally behind a purpose that drives and sustains your efforts. These values will serve as your compass, guiding you through the journey of establishing habits that are not only effective but also deeply aligned with your true self.

Together, let's take the time to explore what truly matters to you and create a path to lasting and meaningful change.

Let's start by thinking about filling your day with joy. What people, things, places, activities, etc. bring you the most joy (think about today but also in the past).

- What aspects of your life bring you the most joy, fulfilment, and satisfaction? Think of the people, the places, the spaces, the activities—think about today and a moment in the past that comes to mind.

- Reflect on a time when you felt truly fulfilled and alive. What were you doing? How can you recreate that sense of fulfilment in your current life today?

- What actions do you currently incorporate into your life that bring you the most joy? No matter how small, focus on the things that really bring you joy!

DID YOU KNOW?

Visualising your future can significantly increase the likelihood of it coming true. Research has shown that when you vividly imagine your goals and dreams, you activate the same neural networks in your brain involved in actual performance, effectively training your mind for positive outcomes. A study by the University of California, Los Angeles (UCLA) found that visualisation techniques can enhance motivation, increase confidence, and improve performance in various tasks.[ix] This mental rehearsal helps you access your positive energy and prepare for challenging moments during motherhood. By consistently visualising your desired future, you create a clear mental roadmap, making navigating obstacles easier and staying focused on nurturing yourself and your family with confidence and calm.

A visualisation
just for you

Take a deep breath, allowing yourself to fully relax in the present moment. As you breathe in, envision a soft, warm light surrounding you, enveloping you in a sense of peace and tranquillity. Feel any tension or worries melting away with each exhale, leaving you feeling light and free. Imagine yourself standing at the edge of a vast, serene lake, surrounded by lush greenery and the gentle sounds of nature. The water is calm and inviting, reflecting the golden rays of the sun above. With each breath you take, feel yourself becoming more grounded and connected to the earth beneath you. Allow the warmth of the sun to envelop you. As you gaze out at the expansive horizon, envision your journey through pregnancy and motherhood stretching out before you like the open waters of the lake. See yourself navigating the waves with grace and confidence, guided by the inner wisdom and strength that resides within you. Visualise your baby nestled safely within your womb, surrounded by love and warmth. Feel your bond growing stronger with each passing moment, a connection transcending time and space.

Now, shift your focus inward and bring your attention to your heart centre. Feel the gentle rhythm of your heartbeat, a constant reminder of the life force that flows through you and sustains you. As you prepare to embark on this sacred journey of motherhood, remember that self-care is not selfish—it is essential. Just as you nourish and care for your growing baby, so too must you nurture and honour yourself. Pregnancy is not just about preparing for your baby's arrival; it's a profound opportunity to connect with yourself on a deeper level. It's a time to explore who you are, what you value, and what brings you joy.

As you journey through pregnancy, see yourself creating habits that will shape your journey into motherhood. These habits are more than just routines; they are the building blocks of your wellbeing. They anchor you, ground you, and give you the strength and resilience to handle whatever journey motherhood may bring. Feel yourself connecting with the growing life within you, nurturing and cherishing the bond between mother and baby. This connection is a powerful reminder of the strength and beauty of your own body and the incredible journey it is capable of.

Allow yourself to expand into this new role, embracing the changes and transformations that pregnancy brings. But amidst the excitement and anticipation, never lose sight of who you are.

Your passions, dreams, and identity are all a vital part of who you are, and they deserve to be honoured and nurtured as you embark on this journey. As you move through each day of pregnancy, remember to pause, breathe, and connect with yourself, whether through gentle movement, quiet reflection, or simply taking a few moments to rest. And just as important as nurturing yourself is surrounding yourself with support.

Your village—whether it's friends, family, or a community of fellow mothers—is there to lift you, to support you, and to remind you that you are never alone on this journey. With this newfound awareness, open your heart to the infinite possibilities that lie ahead. Embrace the joy, the challenges, and the miracles that await you on this extraordinary adventure. When you're ready, slowly bring your awareness back to the present moment, gently wiggle your fingers and toes, and take one final deep breath. As you open your eyes, carry the sense of peace and empowerment you've cultivated with you into the world, knowing that you are capable of embracing the journey of pregnancy and motherhood with grace, courage, and unwavering love for the incredible woman you are.

Your
vision board

Create a vision board that encapsulates your ideal state of wellbeing as you transition into motherhood. This visual representation of your goals and aspirations serves as a tangible reminder of the ideal state of wellbeing you wish to cultivate across mind, body, and soul. By consciously selecting images, words, and symbols that resonate with your deepest values and aspirations, you create a blueprint for the life you wish to lead during pregnancy and beyond.

The process of creating your vision board is an act of self-reflection and intention-setting. Begin by considering what holistic health means to you. What does a confident and fulfilling life look like as you prepare for motherhood? Draw inspiration from those you admire—whether it's the calm presence of a mentor, the nurturing energy of a mother figure, or the vitality of a wellness expert. Reflect on what truly matters to you, be it the ability to nurture your child with love, maintaining your physical health, and/or fostering a resilient and positive mindset. As you gather images, words, and symbols, think about how each element supports your holistic vision. Include representations of physical health, such as nourishing foods, exercise routines, or restful sleep. Incorporate mental wellbeing by selecting quotes or affirmations that promote a positive mindset, resilience, and emotional balance. Don't forget to embrace your spiritual wellbeing, whether through symbols of meditation, creativity, or other practices that connect you to your inner self.

Arrange these elements on your vision board in a way that feels meaningful and inspiring to you. This is your personal guide, so let your intuition lead the way. Once complete, place your vision board in a prominent location where you will see it daily. This constant visual reminder serves not only to motivate you but also to align your actions with your intentions. Each time you glance at your vision board, it will reinforce your commitment to nurturing your mind, body, and soul, guiding you through the inevitable ups and downs of pregnancy and motherhood. By keeping your vision board at the forefront of your daily life, you empower yourself to make conscious choices that support your holistic health. It becomes a source of strength, motivation, and clarity, helping you stay connected to your true self and your goals even when challenges arise. Ultimately, this practice can be a transformative tool in your journey, fostering a deeper sense of wellbeing and fulfilment as you embrace the beautiful, complex path of motherhood.

Once you've had time to create your vision board take a moment to start to define your values.

Are there any words that spring to mind that represent your vision and what's important to you? Defining your values starts to give you a benchmark from which to make decisions and to take action. Feel free to define additional words if these do not resonate.

Circle 3-4 words that really resonate with you (these must be inspired by the things that bring you joy). These start to define what's important to you, in short, your values.

Vitality – Authenticity – Energy – Courage – Gratitude – Respect – Empathy – Simplicity – Resilience – Calm – Generosity – Growth – Love – Balance – Adventure – Creativity – Harmony – Independence – Family – Health – Joy – Kindness – Connection – Patience - Self-discipline – Success – Adventure – Exploration – Wisdom – Optimism - Open mindedness – Freedom – Security – Innovation – Justice – Spirituality – Sustainability – Trust – Unity – Honesty – Purpose – Peace

Label them on the diagram below:

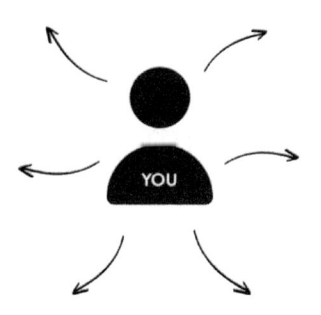

What does wellbeing *mean to you?*

Wellbeing is more than just a set of goals or metrics; it's a deeply personal journey towards feeling truly joyful and aligned with your core values. It's about challenging old narratives that define success and health in narrow terms and embracing a broader perspective instead. Wellbeing should not be solely about achieving specific outcomes like losing weight, but rather about understanding and pursuing the deeper reasons behind those goals. For instance, the desire to shed a few pounds might stem from greater motivation, such as wanting the energy and strength to play with your children as they grow. Reframing wellbeing in this way allows our efforts to align with our values, leading to a more fulfilling and purpose-driven journey.

It is this core change that has enlightened me on why my fitness regime went completely out the window when my children arrived. It's because my why was not strong enough. It was not enough for me to want to stay slim, fit into a size eight, or run a 5km run in twenty-two minutes. I needed a bigger why. As my journey has progressed through motherhood, I have had to focus more on my why. Being fit and healthy truly brings me joy and I love the feeling of going for a walk in nature and listening to music or a podcast and most of all I love knowing that I can be active with my boys as they continue to grow. I wish I had clarity on my whys before I became a mother!

Think about the following questions to understand what wellbeing means to you and what is driving your thoughts and actions:

- What aspects of wellbeing resonate most with you right now? Why are these important?
- How do your values and priorities shape your understanding of wellbeing?
- What does a fulfilling and joyful life look like to you?
- How do you want your wellbeing journey to influence your daily life and relationships?
- How do your achievements and goals align with your wellbeing?
- Finish the sentence: Wellbeing is—

Weekly
reflections

As you become aware of your vision and values, now is the time to start to think about how you can align your actions accordingly. Regular positive self-reflection every week empowers you to recognise and celebrate your progress, no matter how small. It fosters a mindset of growth and positivity, which is crucial for navigating the transformative journey of motherhood. Each week, think about the following:

Wins of the Week: Celebrate your aligned achievements, however small they might be. Example: Took a ten-minute walk in nature each day.

Strengths Demonstrated: Identify and list personal strengths that you demonstrated. Example: Patience, Commitment, Resilience.

Gratitude: Write about things you are grateful for. Example: Grateful for the support of my partner or friends.

Reflection and Intentions: Are there any ways in which you can continue to take more aligned actions? Write down any early ideas or focus points for the upcoming week.

A Quick Recap

This chapter focuses on the transformative journey into motherhood, emphasising the importance of embracing change and grounding yourself in your core values. We explore how values drive actions, the powerful "think-do-feel" model, and understanding your deeper "why" as you navigate this new chapter of life. By aligning your mindset and behaviours with your intentions, you can foster a sense of balance and empowerment throughout pregnancy and motherhood.

Key Points:

- **Embracing change:** This is crucial for personal growth and navigating the transition into motherhood.
- **The Think-Do-Feel model:** This encourages a proactive approach to sticking to healthy habits that are more aligned to your values.
- **Living by your core values:** Identifying and living by your core values helps drive meaningful actions aligned with your wellbeing.
- **Understanding your why:** This is essential for staying motivated and maintaining a sense of purpose.

Chapter Three

DEBUNKING MOTHER-HOOD MYTHS

Motherhood is often surrounded by a cloud of myths and misconceptions that can create unnecessary pressure and unrealistic expectations. These myths can make you doubt your instincts, question your decisions, and feel like you're falling short. Believing these myths can be a significant barrier to thriving as you transition into motherhood. It's essential to understand and come to terms with the fact that these myths will likely be ever-present after becoming a mother. However, we have the power to choose not to believe them and to create the tools required to help overcome any negative thoughts that arise because of these myths. **Prepare to debunk these myths and empower yourself with the truth, paving the way for a healthier, happier journey through motherhood that is fully aligned with your authentic self!**

> **BECOMING A MOTHER LEAVES NO WOMAN AS IT FOUND HER.**
>
> *Nikki McCahon*

BALANCE

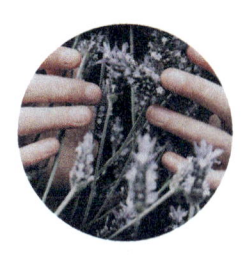

"I will be able to juggle everything, because I've been told I can." One common myth about motherhood is that the goal is to achieve perfect balance. Balance is often an elusive ideal. It's not about evenly distributing your time among all your responsibilities but rather about being comfortable with prioritising what's important at a certain point in time. Embrace the ebb and flow of your daily life, and recognise that some days you'll need to prioritise self-care over ironing the clothes. By accepting this, you'll find a more realistic and fulfilling approach to managing your time and energy, ensuring that you focus on what truly matters and not trying to do it all.

TIME

"I shouldn't ask for help; I should be able to handle everything on my own." The myth that there will always be enough time for everything is just that—a myth. Motherhood brings new demands that inevitably reduces the time available for yourself. Effective time management becomes crucial. Learn to prioritise your tasks and ask for help when possible. Finding your village—a supportive community of family, friends, and fellow mums—can provide much-needed assistance and companionship. Remember, it's about making the most of your time rather than striving for an impossible ideal & trying to fit everything into the time you have.

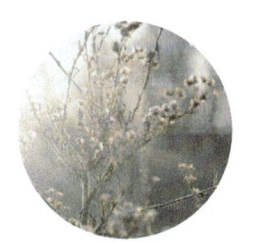

MUM GUILT

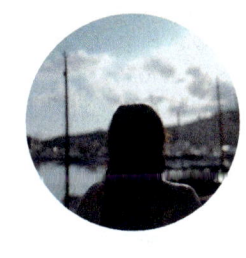

"I shouldn't take time for myself; my baby needs me 24/7." Mum guilt is a relentless companion that many mothers face. The truth is, it's not going anywhere. Instead of trying to eliminate it, acknowledge its presence and let it go. Understand that feeling guilty doesn't make you a bad mother—it's a common emotion stemming from the immense love and responsibility you feel. Accepting mum guilt as a natural part of motherhood can help you move past it and focus on what truly matters: nurturing yourself and your family.

SUPERMUM SYNDROME

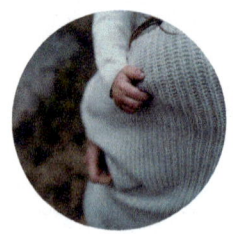

"I should instinctively know how to be a perfect mother." The myth of the "super mum" suggests that you should be able to do it all: perfect parenting, maintaining a spotless home, thriving in your career, and staying socially active. This myth sets unrealistic expectations and can lead to burnout. It's essential to recognise that no one can do it all, and trying to live up to this ideal can be detrimental to your wellbeing. Embrace your imperfections and understand that seeking help, taking breaks and prioritising what's truly important to you in any given period of time, are signs of strength, not weakness.

COMPARISON

"Everyone else knows what to do—so should I." Every mother's journey is unique, and measuring your experiences against others' highlights only the differences, often leading to feelings of inadequacy. Instead of focusing on how you measure up to others, embrace your path and recognise the strengths and successes in your unique journey. Remember, there is no one-size-fits-all approach to motherhood, and what works for one family may not work for another. Celebrate your individuality and trust that you are the best mother for your child.

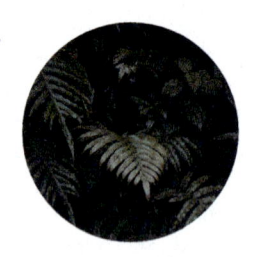

ETERNAL HAPPINESS

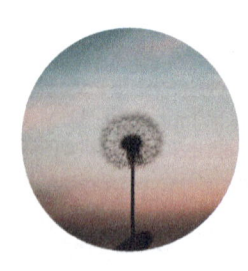

"I'm a bad mother if I don't feel happy and fulfilled all the time." Motherhood is a complex journey filled with highs and lows, and it's expected to experience a range of emotions. Believing that you should always be joyful dismisses the validity of your struggles and can lead to guilt and frustration when you inevitably face challenges. True happiness in motherhood comes from accepting and embracing the full spectrum of emotions, finding joy in small moments, and prioritising your wellbeing. By acknowledging that it's okay to have difficult days, you create space for genuine fulfilment in your life.

BODY BOUNCE BACK

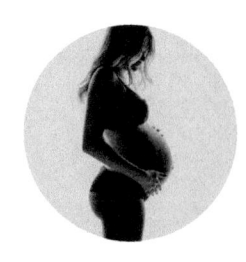

"I need to bounce back to my pre-pregnancy body quickly." The pressure to quickly return to your pre-pregnancy body is a common myth that many new mothers face. However, the reality is that your body has just accomplished something incredible—nurturing and bringing a new life into the world. Rather than rushing to fit into old clothes or meet unrealistic standards, it's important to focus on healing, self-care, and appreciating the strength and resilience of your body. Embrace this new chapter with compassion and patience, knowing that your body will find its own balance in time. Your worth isn't defined by how quickly you "bounce back" but by the love and care you provide for yourself and your baby.

BREASTFEEDING & WEIGHT LOSS

"Breastfeeding will automatically help me lose all the baby weight." The idea that breastfeeding will automatically help you lose all the baby weight is a common misconception. While breastfeeding can burn extra calories and contribute to weight loss for some, it's not a guarantee. Every woman's body responds differently, and many factors, such as metabolism, diet, and overall health, play a role in postpartum weight loss. It's important not to put undue pressure on yourself to shed weight quickly. Instead, focus on nourishing your body to support both your recovery and your baby's growth. Remember, your worth isn't tied to your weight—celebrate your body for the incredible work it's done and be patient with yourself as you heal and adjust to your new role as a mother.

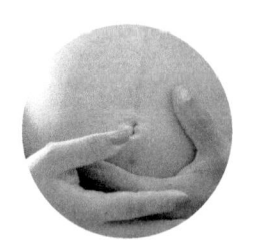

IT STARTS
with love

You're here because you love yourself enough to know that focusing on your health and wellbeing is essential, especially when facing the challenges of motherhood and the myths and misconceptions that come with it. This self-love is the foundation of your journey. By prioritising your health and wellbeing, you're caring for yourself and setting a powerful example for your new baby.

Show yourself love every single day, even amidst the demands of motherhood and the myths that surround us. Remember, nobody is perfect, and it's okay to have moments where you fall off the wagon. The key is to approach these moments with grace and understanding.

Your wellbeing toolkit is here to support you on this incredible journey. It serves as a positive companion, focusing on holistic wellbeing for joy, health, and happiness. This is not about restrictions or what you cannot do; it's about discovering the beautiful practices that work for you and enhance your life.

Loving yourself enough to prioritise your health and wellbeing is one of the most important mindset shifts you can take into motherhood. Embrace the journey of holistic health, and you'll find that it truly is the key to lasting happiness and fulfilment.

A Quick Recap

This chapter dives into some of the myths and misconceptions that often surround motherhood, dispelling unrealistic expectations and pressures that can hold you back. These myths—whether about balance, time, mum guilt, or body image—can make it harder to thrive as a new mother. By recognising these untruths and empowering yourself with the facts, you can let go of unnecessary guilt, embrace imperfections, and focus on what really matters for you and your family.

Key Points:

- **What's a Myth?** Myths about motherhood can lead to unrealistic expectations, making you feel like you're constantly falling short.
- **Common Myths Include:**
    - You must achieve perfect balance.
    - There will always be enough time for everything.
    - Mum guilt means you're failing.
    - You should instinctively know how to be the perfect mum.
    - You need to quickly "bounce back" to your pre-pregnancy body.
- **It Starts with Love:** The foundation of a positive motherhood journey is self-love. By caring for your well-being, you set an example for your baby and build the strength to navigate challenges with grace.

Chapter Four

MOTHER-
HOOD
MINDSET
SHIFTS

As you journey through pregnancy and beyond, you'll find that your emotional landscape is ever-changing - One moment, you might be filled with an overwhelming sense of joy and anticipation; the next, you could ride a wave of uncertainty or unexpected frustration. Embracing this emotional ebb and flow is essential to preparing for motherhood. By acknowledging that these feelings are not only expected but also a crucial aspect of this transformative time, you are already taking the first step towards creating a supportive wellbeing toolkit for yourself.

This chapter will gently guide you through some mindset shifts and practical things you can start to work on today to provide you with the foundations to handle these emotions if, and when, they arise during motherhood and enhancing your focus on the **Pause** and **Expand** wellbeing levers.

> **PEACE. IT DOES NOT MEAN TO BE IN A PLACE WHERE THERE IS NO NOISE, TROUBLE OR HARD WORK. IT MEANS TO BE IN THE MIDST OF THOSE THINGS AND STILL BE CALM IN YOUR HEART.**
>
> *Anonymous*

The highs & lows
of parenting

The emotional rollercoaster of motherhood can bring up feelings you never knew you had, ranging from intense love and joy to frustration, stress, and anxiety. Sleepless nights and new responsibilities can feel overwhelming, and whilst the deep bond with your child can offer strength and comfort, it is the strength within yourself that will enable you to ride the waves as and when they come.

It's essential to acknowledge that these feelings are not just emotional; they also manifest physically. Stress, for example, triggers the release of cortisol, a hormone that prepares your body to deal with challenges. However, when cortisol levels remain high for long periods of time, as they often do during the demands of early motherhood, this can lead to several negative health effects. High cortisol levels can disrupt sleep, weaken the immune system, and even affect your mood and mental clarity, creating a cycle of stress that can be difficult to break.

Moments of joy in simple interactions can reframe mindsets, whilst feelings of loneliness and anxiety are natural but manageable with support and self-care. Developing tools and techniques to manage stress and its effects on your body is crucial. Practicing mindfulness, engaging in regular physical activity, and ensuring you have a support system in place can help keep cortisol levels in check, promoting both emotional and physical well-being.

Remember, there is no right way to feel during this time. It's unpredictable and, at times, intense, but by becoming aware of your emotional patterns and building the tools and techniques to help you work through them throughout pregnancy, you'll find a newfound strength and resilience within yourself. Preparing these tools in advance not only supports your mental health but also helps your body cope better with the physical demands of motherhood.

Here, we look at some of the most common motherhood mindset shifts and offer some tools to get started to draw your awareness to them and build strength in your mindset whilst you journey through pregnancy. These tools focus mostly on our Pause and Expand levers offering the opportunity to slow down, reflect and find ways to tap into your light. These practices will build strength in how you think and support your transition to motherhood.

Some mindset shifts may already feel relevant to you, whilst others may not resonate yet. Pick one or two that you relate to the most at this stage and work through the activities over a three-week period. Even if the remaining mindset shifts feel distant, being aware of them and understanding the tools to manage them is key, so continue working through them throughout your pregnancy. Your ability to manage stress, and your fluctuating emotions, will grow stronger enabling you to embrace the highs and navigate the lows with greater ease.

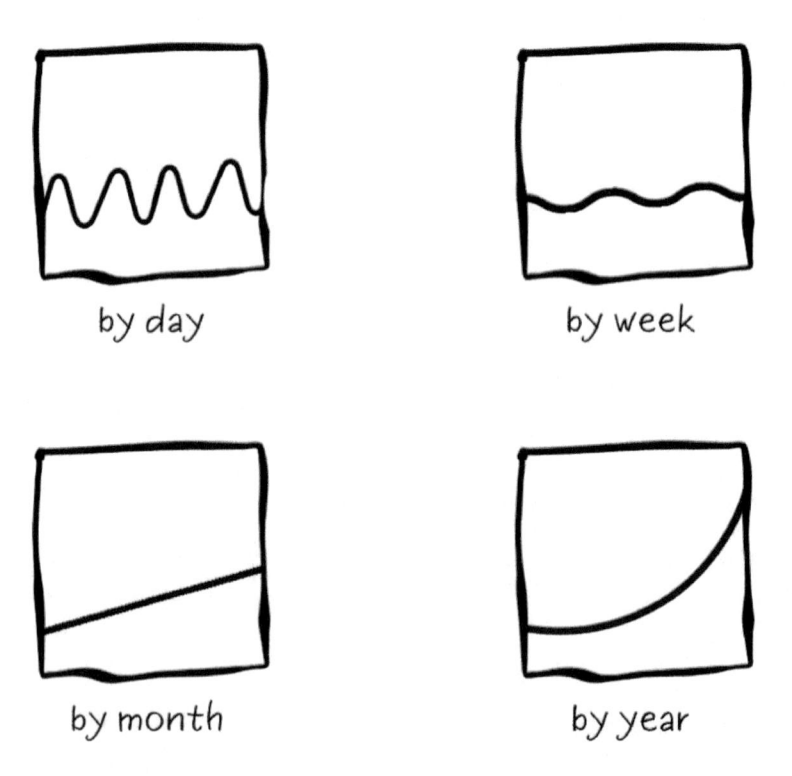

by day

by week

by month

by year

MINDSET *shifts*

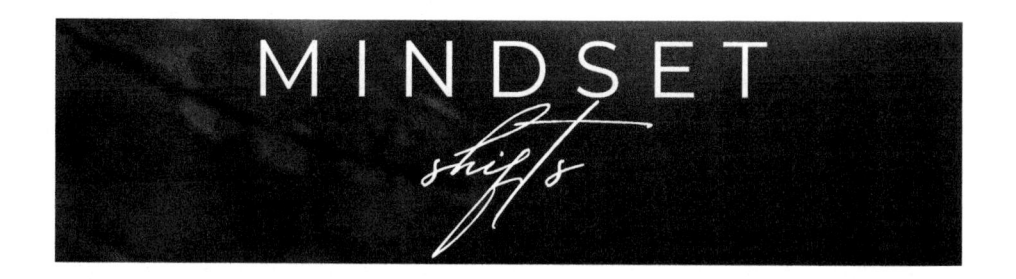

NEWFOUND PURPOSE

Before motherhood, priorities might centre around personal and professional goals. Whilst these should continue to be important the real why behind a mother's actions becomes all too apparent and can sometimes do a complete 180. Understanding your why and your vision and being clear about this will help you navigate the change with confidence and conviction. Living in alignment with your purpose acts as your North Star. It can provide you with guidance when you feel like you're going off course.

Before becoming a mother, I thought I needed to a certain weight to look good. Now, I know this was not enough to keep me motivated to stay fit after becoming a mother, and that's the reason I struggled to keep my fitness routine consistent after having my babies. It took me years to understand that whilst I have always loved being fit and healthy, I needed a deep-rooted reason to prioritise it over other things and to ignore the mum guilt whenever I chose to go for a run instead of be home with the family. I now know that I want to be fit and healthy so that I can easily pick up my boys and play sports and games with them whilst they grow older. Now, when I have to choose to get up earlier to go out for a run or not, I come back to that why again and again, and it helps me align my decision making.

Things to Try:

Spend a few minutes each day reflecting on your motivations and goals. Repeatedly ask yourself why. Initially, what we feel we need and want can be somewhat superficial. But if you keep asking why, you will start to get underneath the surface of your deep motivations. It's this that will then drive you forwards. The why might change as you move into motherhood, and that's fine; the main thing is to start this practice so that it becomes a habit and can help guide you if you become lost or overwhelmed.

EMBRACE GOOD ENOUGH

In a world that often emphasises perfection, motherhood teaches the invaluable lesson of embracing good enough. The pressure to be the perfect parent can be overwhelming, but striving for perfection can lead to unnecessary stress and unrealistic expectations. Instead, understanding that being a good enough mother is acceptable and healthy can be liberating. This mindset allows mothers to focus on what truly matters—the love, care, and presence they provide. Children thrive on love and connection, not perfection, and recognising this can help mothers navigate their journey with more confidence and peace.

For me, this was a significant challenge—being a serial perfectionist. I found it difficult when my son's nap times didn't match what the book predicted (I know, it sounds extreme) or when the house was constantly messy with toys, laundry, and unmade beds. I had to come to terms with the fact that motherhood isn't about achieving perfection; otherwise, I risked burning out. Now, my house doesn't always look perfect but I'm at peace with it. If you struggle with perfectionism, it might be worth working through this during pregnancy.

Things to Try:

Keep a journal listing three things you did well each day, no matter how small. This practice will help you focus on your strengths rather than perceived shortcomings.

RELEASE CONTROL

Motherhood quickly teaches that control is an illusion. From unpredictable sleep patterns to sudden illnesses, a mother's plans often need to be flexible. Releasing control means embracing the unpredictability of life with a baby and learning to adapt. This shift fosters resilience and teaches mothers to find stability amidst chaos. Accepting that not everything can be planned or controlled allows for a more relaxed and responsive approach to parenting and releases the pressure we, as mothers, can sometimes put on ourselves.

This was a profound lesson for me. Becoming a mother at thirty-three meant I had ample time to focus solely on myself. I enjoyed complete control over my life, from work and travel to my social life. Then came my children—an experience where control seems almost non-existent, starting with something as basic as the birth plan. A birth plan can only serve as an intention; ultimately, you must surrender and let things unfold as they will.

What's intriguing is that whilst I once had control over every aspect of my life, I never had control over my emotions. And the reality is that the only thing we can actually control is how we respond to the events around us, not the events themselves. To work on accepting this and releasing control, try the following exercises.

Things to Try:

Identify a situation where you feel a strong need to control the outcome. Write it down and reflect on why you feel this way. Consider the aspects of this situation you can and cannot control. List them separately. Focus on the aspects you can control, particularly your responses and reactions. Write down how you can positively influence these aspects.

Practice mindfulness or meditation for a few minutes each day. During this time, acknowledge your feelings and gently remind yourself that whilst you can't control everything, you can choose how to respond.

End with a daily affirmation: "I release the need to control and embrace the power of my responses." Repeat this affirmation whenever you feel the urge to control.

CULTIVATE CURIOSITY

Change is inevitable in motherhood, and embracing curiosity can be a powerful tool. Getting curious about oneself and the baby can transform challenges into opportunities for learning and growth. Curiosity fosters a mindset of continuous learning, making the journey of motherhood an adventure rather than a series of obstacles. Motherhood often acts as a mirror, reflecting a mother's strengths and flaws - It's a journey of self-discovery where personal limitations and virtues become more apparent. This reflection can be challenging but also offers growth and self-improvement opportunities. Embracing this aspect of motherhood with humility and openness can lead to profound personal development and a deeper understanding of oneself.

Things to Try:

Dedicate time each week to learning something new about yourself. Keep a journal of these observations and insights without judgement and enjoy the process of discovery.

EMBRACE POSITIVE ENERGY

Motherhood will test patience and endurance, making it crucial to find ways to engage in positive energy. Practices like gratitude journaling can help mothers focus on the positive aspects of their daily experiences. Reflecting on small victories, joyful moments, and the love shared with their child can uplift spirits and provide motivation. Cultivating a positive mindset helps navigate motherhood's ups and downs with grace and resilience.

Reconnecting with activities that once brought you joy is one powerful way to foster personal growth and positive energy. Engaging in hobbies like singing, hiking, reading, or creative writing can help you enter a state of flow where you're deeply absorbed in the activity and lose track of time. This state not only enhances performance but also leads to a profound sense of fulfilment and happiness. For example, studies have shown that creative activities such as painting or playing music can reduce stress and increase overall wellbeing. Regularly making time for these activities helps you stay connected to your interests, maintain your sense of self, and combat feelings of stagnation or burnout. It gives you a sense of purpose beyond parenting, providing positive energy and fulfilment.

Equally, exploring new interests or learning new skills can significantly impact your mental wellbeing. Engaging in novel activities or discovering new places and spaces helps stimulate the brain and prevents life from feeling monotonous. Research indicates that learning new skills can enhance cognitive function, increase neuroplasticity (the brain's ability to adapt and grow), and improve overall mental health. For instance, one study found that learning new things, such as a new language or musical instrument, can improve memory and cognitive flexibility.[x] Finding new hobbies or pursuing new experiences keeps your mind active and engaged, creating a sense of excitement and preventing the feeling of being stuck in a repetitive routine.

Things to Try:

Each day, think about engaging in an activity that brings you into a state of flow. The key here is to not worry about how long you're doing it; even five minutes is great!

Then use one or more of these prompts to write down three things you are grateful for. This practice will help shift your focus from challenges to positive experiences, fostering a more uplifting and resilient mindset:

- What small moment today brought you positive energy or a state of flow?
- Think about a small victory you achieved today: completing a task, handling a challenging situation, or simply making it through the day.
- What is one thing you appreciate about yourself today? Reflect on a quality or action that you value.
- Identify a simple pleasure that brought you joy today. It could be a warm cup of coffee, a beautiful moment with nature, or a quiet moment of self-care.
- Consider a challenge you faced today. What did it teach you, and how did you grow from it?

MR COMPARISON

Comparison can be an unwelcome companion on the journey of motherhood. As a mother, it's easy to fall into the trap of comparing not just your child's milestones—crawling, walking, eating solids, or sleeping through the night—with those of other children but also comparing yourself to other mothers. You might find yourself wondering who is losing weight the quickest, who has more help, or who seems to have it all together. This constant comparison can create unnecessary stress and self doubt, often amplified by your inner critic, who might whisper: I'm not doing enough, or others are handling it better. Despite your best efforts, the urge to measure your progress and situation against others is nearly inevitable. Building mental resilience and managing your inner critic is crucial in navigating this aspect of motherhood. Focus on your unique journey and celebrate your individual achievements without the weight of comparison or self-judgement. Regularly engaging in this exercise can shift your mindset from comparison and self-criticism to appreciation and self-compassion, building resilience and embracing the unique path of your motherhood journey.

Things to Try:

- **Create a Celebration Journal:** Each day, write down one thing you appreciate or celebrate about your journey, regardless of how it compares to others.
- **Challenge Your Inner Critic:** When you notice negative self-talk or critical thoughts, write them down. Then, counter these thoughts with positive affirmations or evidence of your strengths.

EMBRACE TIME

Often, becoming a mother brings a profound shift in how we perceive and manage time. It can feel like our children are in control of our schedules, leaving us with little ownership over our own time. This shift can lead to feelings of frustration and helplessness.

However, it's important to reframe this perception and recognise that whilst the demands of motherhood are significant, we still have the power to manage our time effectively and make space for ourselves. Embracing a mindset of flexibility and intentionality can help us regain control and find balance within the new rhythms of our lives.

Having my first baby at thirty-three made it challenging to accept that my entire life now revolved around a tiny human, and I felt increasingly out of touch with my own needs. However, I realised this was a mistake. I needed to incorporate activities into my daily routine that were for me, not just for my newborn, but I honestly didn't know how. After some time, I realised that intentionally carving out time for myself every day (even just twenty minutes to have a bath) provided a sense of anticipation and helped me maintain a focus on my own wellbeing, whilst reducing any build-up of resentment.

Things to Try:

- List your daily tasks (one of which should include self-care) and prioritise them. Focus on completing the most critical tasks first, allowing flexibility for unexpected changes.
- Allocate a specific length of time for different activities. For example, set aside forty minutes for household chores or twenty minutes for self-care. It doesn't matter what time these happen; just stick to these time blocks as closely as possible to create a structured routine.
- At the end of each week, reflect on what worked well and what didn't. Adjust your schedule as needed to better align with your needs and priorities.

JOY IN THE SMALL THINGS

Motherhood simplifies life, focusing on its most basic yet profoundly essential aspects. As you transition into this new phase, fostering a mindset that finds joy in the small things becomes vital. Whether it's your morning coffee or a beautiful sunset, you can start cultivating this mindset even before the baby arrives, easing the transition into motherhood and allowing you to embrace and cherish the richness of everyday experiences with a renewed sense of purpose and joy.

I used to believe that joy came from significant events in life—like a two-week holiday by the sea or an annual birthday party. But I've come to realise that I was overlooking the small, everyday moments that bring the most delight. Now, I find joy in the simple pleasures: the sunrise each morning, a quiet coffee before the day begins, and reading for twenty minutes before bed. This shift has transformed my experience of motherhood, too.

It's not just about the exciting outings but also the cosy moments, like snuggling on the sofa and watching a silly movie with my kids. In the end, it's these positive feelings and shared memories that truly matter. Try the following activity to work on refocusing the mind to enjoy the smaller joys in life.

Things to Try:

Try a Dopamine Detox - this is a break from the constant stimulation and temptations that surround us; the social media feed, the video game, the crisps whilst binging on Netflix. These habits provide a quick pick-me-up, a surge of motivation, and a fleeting sense of pleasure. Yet, they come at a cost—they wire our brains for instant gratification. A Dopamine detox, often referred to as a "dopamine fast," is a method aimed at reducing overstimulation from these activities and its goal is to reset the brain's rewards system. In short, it can be a positive way to break bad habits and help us find joy in more natural things. Before you set out on a 'dopamine detox', seek to be clear on the habits you would like to change. Ultimately, a dopamine detox must be a personalised one so you must also decide what your fasting periods will be (times that these activities are off-limits). And because it takes about 66 days, on average, to build a new habit, the best approach would be to aim for a longer detox to help you wire your brain for joyful habits. The aim is to take charge of your impulses and reassess priorities for a more joyful way of living. List the changes you'd like to make below:

SWAP OUT	SWAP IN

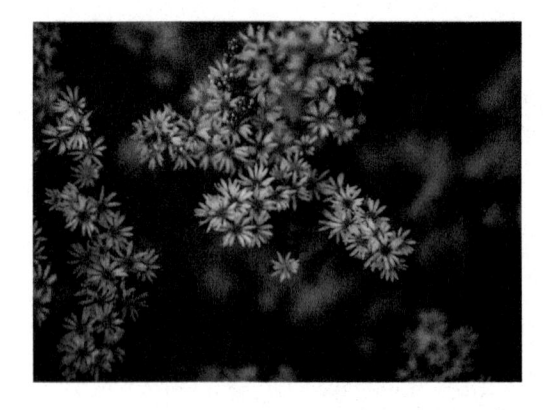

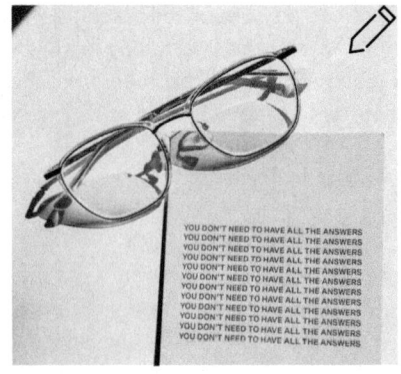

The art of
morning pages

As you can see, journaling is a powerful tool to help you connect with your inner self and make sense of your emotions. Set aside a few minutes each day to write down your thoughts and feelings. This practice can provide clarity, release pent-up emotions, and become a cherished time of self-reflection. Morning Pages are three pages of longhand, stream-of-consciousness writing, done first thing in the morning. *There is no wrong way to do Morning Pages*– they are not high art. They are not even writing. They are about anything and everything that crosses your mind and are for your eyes only. Morning Pages provoke, clarify, comfort, cajole, prioritise and synchronise the day at hand. Do not overthink Morning Pages: just put three pages of anything on the page and then do three more pages tomorrow.

Here are Some Prompts to Get You Started:

- How am I feeling today, both physically and emotionally?
- What is the most prominent emotion I'm experiencing right now?
- What thoughts or events have triggered this emotion?
- How can I be kind to myself in this moment?
- What am I grateful for today?

It all begins with love – specifically, love for yourself. Embracing self-love is the foundation upon which all other forms of love and fulfilment are built. By prioritising self-care and self-compassion now, you create a strong foundation for a positive experience and a healthier transition into motherhood, enabling you to give and receive love more authentically and generously.

DID YOU KNOW?

Learning to use your breath to pause, centre yourself, and become more present is a powerful practice, especially during the intense transition into motherhood. But no breath is made equal! One thing's for sure, we have lost the art of breathing well. And while we spend money and time searching for external things that can help us stay calm, focused, or energised, we have the power within to guide our mood and feelings.

Breathwork helps anchor you in the moment, reduce stress, and foster a sense of calm amidst the chaos. Focusing on your breath can create a brief but effective pause in your day, allowing you to reset and approach challenges with a clearer mind.

Start incorporating this practice by setting aside just five minutes each morning and see how this transforms the way you feel:

Visualise a square as you breathe in four equal parts: inhale, hold, exhale, hold. Start by inhaling deeply through your nose for a count of four. Hold your breath for a count of four. Exhale slowly and completely through your mouth for a count of four. Hold your breath again for a count of four. Repeat this cycle for several rounds, maintaining a steady and controlled rhythm.

Box Breathing helps to regulate your nervous system, bringing about a state of calm and balance and is an excellent technique to use during stressful moments.

Inspiring Your Mind
Toolkit

Reflecting on all the different exercises, which ones could work for you to start incorporating into your daily/weekly life? One or two will be plenty. Take the wellbeing toolkit template and fill it out. Remember, try these out for three weeks; if they just aren't working, then come back and revisit some of the other exercises to see if something else might work better for you. Remain curious; nothing is set in stone, and learn about what resonates with you over time and tweak your toolkit to fit your lifestyle.

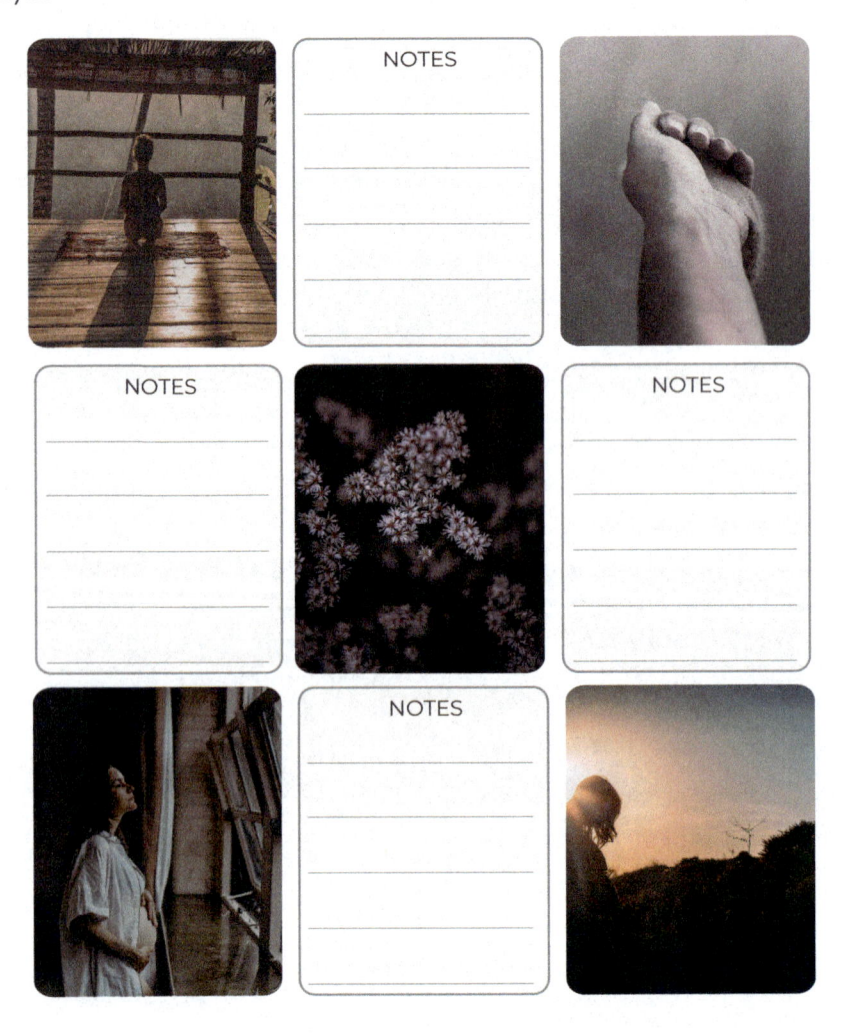

NOTES

NOTES

NOTES

NOTES

A Quick Recap

In this chapter, we focused on the importance of nurturing a positive mindset during pregnancy and as you transition into motherhood by tackling some of the most significant mindset shifts we, as mothers, might experience. By integrating practices that help you **pause** and **expand**, you can find moments to be present and maintain a strong sense of self amidst the changes and challenges of motherhood.

Key Points:

- **Pause for Presence:** Incorporate daily pauses to ground yourself and stay present, allowing you to experience and appreciate the journey of pregnancy and motherhood fully.
- **Expand for Growth:** Embrace opportunities for mental and emotional expansion, helping you to grow and adapt positively to new experiences.
- **Mindset Practices:** Establish consistent practices that support a positive mindset, such as mindfulness, meditation, or journaling, to navigate the transition with resilience and grace.
- **Morning Pages:** Spend some time each morning writing your morning pages and see how this gives you a sense of liberation and freedom.
- **The Power of Breath:** We have lost the art of breathing properly, but there are many ways to use the breath to help to centre us. Practise Box Breathing and see how it helps you feel more calm.

Chapter Five

THE BODY - A MARVEL OF NATURE

We've spent some time focusing on the mind and identifying practices that can help to build mental strength, confidence, and resilience. But the mind is not disconnected from the body (or the soul).

Emerging research highlights the brain-gut connection and how the health of our gut microbiome affects mental and physical wellbeing.[xi] By focusing on a balanced diet rich in nutrients, you can support your gut health and, in turn, enhance your overall mood and energy. Integrating foods that nourish both body and mind helps harness the full potential of your body's recovery and adaptation during this time, ensuring a healthier and more vibrant transition into motherhood.

Pregnancy also offers a wonderful opportunity to become truly in tune with your physical body—to understand the marvel of the female body and to work together with it to stay fit, healthy, and strong during pregnancy, which will help to promote a more natural recovery in place of the unnecessary pressure to bounce back quickly.

Here, we focus on the wellbeing levers of **Food** and **Move** and offer insight and practices that can be adopted during pregnancy so that you can support your body in its ongoing transformation. These proactive steps not only prepare you for the physical demands of childbirth and postpartum recovery but also set a solid foundation for long-term wellbeing.

> **REST IS NOT THE ABSENCE OF ACTIVITY BUT THE PRESENCE OF PEACE.**

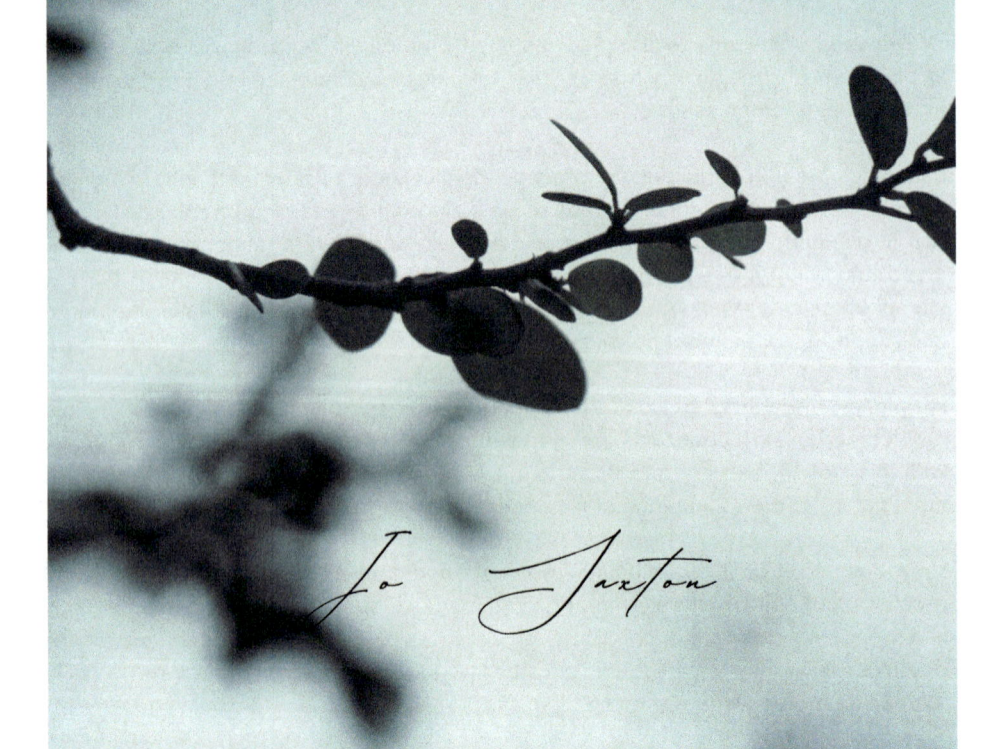

Jo Saxton

OPTIMISING
how we eat

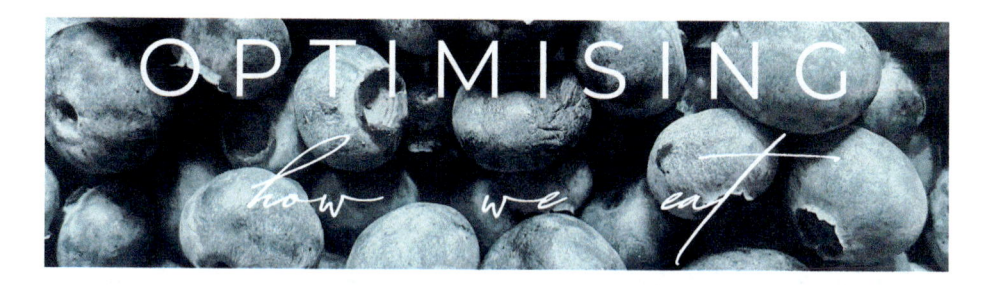

MOOD-BOOSTING MEALS

Eating isn't just about satisfying hunger—it's a great way to support your emotional wellbeing. The foods you choose can significantly impact how you feel, influencing everything from your energy levels to your ability to manage stress. By starting to think about what you eat as a tool for nurturing your mood, you can make choices that fuel your body and uplift your mind. Whether incorporating calming ingredients to help you unwind or energising foods to keep you focused and positive, mindful eating can become a crucial part of your self-care routine.

Certain foods, like those rich in omega-3 fatty acids, magnesium, and B vitamins, can promote a sense of calm, whilst others, such as leafy greens, nuts, and seeds, can help energise you naturally. By focusing on these nutrient-dense ingredients, you can create meals that satisfy your hunger and support your mental and emotional health. Thinking about how you can start to prepare these meals at home (rather than eating out or opting for home delivery) is also crucial for health because it allows you to control the ingredients and cooking methods, ensuring meals are nutritious and free from excessive additives and unhealthy fats. By preparing your meals, you can focus on whole foods, balanced nutrition, and portion control, all essential for your wellbeing and that of your baby. This might feel daunting initially, but building up a bank of easy, quick, yet healthy recipes during pregnancy will make it much easier to continue as you transition into motherhood.

Things to Try:

The ingredients in these lists have powerful properties that impact how you feel. Starting to explore and understand recipes that incorporate mood-boosting ingredients can be transformative for your overall wellbeing. For instance, opting for herbal teas or lemon water instead of caffeinated drinks can reduce anxiety, helping you feel more balanced throughout the day.

Enjoy the journey of discovery whilst you have the time during pregnancy, switch out your cupboard stores to reflect the new, healthy recipes you discover, and maybe set up a recurring delivery every week so your habits can continue into motherhood. There are many wonderful recipe books nowadays, online resources, and kitchen appliances that can support your journey to healthier, mood-boosting eating.

Try to reduce caffeine late in the day and introduce more fibre, fermented foods, and Omega 3s into your diet. Here are some ideas to focus on for different meals:

- Breakfast: Eggs, Oats, Berries or Bran
- Snacks: Kimchi, Almonds, Carrots, Apples and Bananas
- Lunch: Salads with pearl barley, Buckwheat, Walnuts and Beans
- Dinner: Meals with Sweet Potatoes, Brown Rice, Fish rich in Omega 3s, Artichokes
- Desserts: Focus on Plain Yoghurt, Berries and Pears

CALMING INGREDIENTS

The ingredients suggested below have been proven to support the reduction of anxiety in the body. Explore recipes where you can start to incorporate some or all of these ingredients into your meals. Enjoy!

1. If you have a sweet tooth or you really need your sweet fix then head for the **dark chocolate**. Aim for 70% cocoa or higher for less sugar content

2. For something sweet **go for fruit first**, specifically, bananas, blueberries and citrus fruits

3. When needing a mid morning or afternoon snack, pick **roasted almonds or snacks that contain nuts or seeds** such as Chia Seeds, Quinoa or pumpkin seeds

4. For cold drinks, try some fruit infused water or for something hot try **green tea or chamomile**.

5. **Add spices to food and drinks** such as turmeric (to which you should add black pepper to activate the benefits of the turmeric) or ginger - Spices with both antioxidant and anti-anxiety properties

6. For protein fixes, focus on lean meats (turkey, chicken), oily fish (salmon), eggs or tofu - The high level of protein makes tofu a good alternative to animal-derived meat

7. For dairy intake, try to focus on **plain yoghurt or Kefir** - the more fermented the better!

8. Try to increase the amount of veg in your meals - including **artichokes, kale, spinach, beets, broccoli and Kimchi**

ENERGISING INGREDIENTS

The ingredients suggested below have been proven to contain energising properties to lift the mood. Explore recipes where you can start to incorporate some or all of these ingredients into your meals. Enjoy!

1. If you have a sweet tooth or you really need your sweet fix then head for **dates or dried apricots**. These are high in natural sugar.

2. For something sweet **go for fruit first**, specifically, bananas, blueberries and watermelon

3. When needing a mid morning snack, pick **roasted almonds or snacks that contain nuts or seeds** (Chia Seeds, Quinoa, pumpkin seeds)

4. Mint has been shown to be effective at giving you a boost of energy. While peppermint doesn't contain any caffeine or stimulants, it can help to increase alertness, focus, and energy.

5. **Focus on wholegrains, nuts, seeds and oats** for longer lasting energy boosting properties.

6. For protein fixes, focus on lean meats (turkey, chicken), oily fish (salmon), eggs or tofu - The high level of protein makes tofu a good alternative to animal-derived meat

7. For dairy intake, try to focus on **plain yoghurt or Kefir** - the more fermented the better.

8. **Leafy greens and green veggies** are filled with nutrients and power our health. Dark leafy greens, for example, are rich in vitamins A, C, E, and K as well as the B-vitamins essential to converting food into usable energy. Look for avocado, kale, spinach and broccoli.

DID YOU KNOW?

Food and mood are strongly connected.

The ingredients you consume can significantly impact your emotional wellbeing. This relationship between your gut and brain, known as the gut-brain axis, highlights how your eating influences your feelings. Nutrient-rich foods like fruits, vegetables, whole grains, and lean proteins can boost mood, improve mental clarity, and reduce stress. On the other hand, processed foods and high sugar intake can lead to mood swings, anxiety, and sluggishness. By making mindful food choices, you're nourishing your body and supporting a happier, healthier mind. For example, have you heard of the MIND Diet, inspired by a Mediterranean diet that promotes brain health? This diet is rich in brain-boosting foods like leafy greens, berries, nuts, and whole grains. You can think about introducing more of the following into your diet:

- Green Leafy Vegetables: Spinach, Broccoli
- Nuts
- Berries
- Beans and Lentils
- Whole Grains: Oats, Quinoa, Brown Rice
- Fatty Fish, Salmon
- And don't forget to cook with olive oil and oil full of heart-healthy fats that also have anti-inflammatory properties.

ALIGN TO YOUR CIRCADIAN RHYTHMS

Aligning your eating habits with your circadian rhythm—your body's natural sleep-wake cycle—can significantly improve your health and energy levels. Eating in tune with your circadian rhythm involves aligning your mealtimes with your body's natural biological clock, which regulates various physiological processes, including metabolism, digestion, and energy levels. Our bodies are designed to follow a daily cycle influenced by light and dark, which impacts when we're most efficient at processing food.

Research shows that eating earlier in the day when our metabolism is more active, can improve digestion, energy levels, and even weight management.[xii] Breakfast and lunch could be your more substantial meals, with dinner being lighter and eaten earlier in the evening. Late-night eating, when the body is winding down, can disrupt digestion and contribute to weight gain, as our bodies are less efficient at processing food at this time.

Eating in sync with your circadian rhythm helps to regulate blood sugar levels, maintain a healthy weight, and support overall wellbeing. By paying attention to the timing of your meals, you can better support your body's natural cycles, leading to improved health and vitality.

I personally set off on the wrong foot with this one; eating muffins in the middle of the night whilst trying to breastfeed meant I put on more weight after giving birth than throughout the whole pregnancy—yikes! And it took me some time to reverse the bad habit once the sleep deprivation started to set in.

Once you become a mother, this can sometimes go completely out the window, especially in the first few months when you are up overnight feeding the baby every two hours. But establishing a cyclical eating pattern, which might get thrown off course initially, is a skill you can return to once things settle down and will promote a more natural recovery postpartum.

Things to Try:

Instead of reaching for a snack out of habit or fatigue, at critical meal and snacking times throughout the day, ask yourself questions that help you become more aware of your body, for example, "Am I hungry now?" or "How hungry am I?".

These simple questions can help you distinguish between true hunger and emotional eating, which often occurs when we're tired or stressed. By tuning into your body's needs and eating in harmony with your circadian rhythm, you can avoid the temptation to reach for quick fixes like sugary snacks when exhaustion sets in, particularly once your baby arrives.

Try adopting the Japanese art, Hara Hachi Bu. This teaching advises people to eat until they are 80 percent full rather than eating until they are completely full. It's a crucial part of the Okinawan diet associated with longevity and good health. By stopping at 80 percent fullness, the idea is to avoid overeating and promote a balanced and healthy lifestyle.

SWEET SWAP

Reducing your intake of sugary foods is essential for overall health. Excessive sugar consumption can lead to energy crashes, weight gain, and increased risk of chronic diseases like diabetes. Sugary foods and drinks, including fruit juices and highly processed snacks and meals, can also contribute to unhealthy cravings and eating habits. By making these changes during pregnancy, you'll set a solid foundation for healthier eating habits that can benefit you and your baby in the long run.

And if you're worried about cutting out sweet food completely, remember that your taste buds regenerate themselves roughly every 1-2 weeks, which is why people might experience a shift in taste preferences after consistently eating different foods for a relatively short period of time.

Things to Try:

If your go-to breakfast is a sugary cereal (and yes, most cereals are full of sugar), try replacing your cereal with a savoury breakfast. No time? An avocado with brown toast is quick and tasty. Try to focus on incorporating more whole foods into your breakfast to help stabilise blood sugar levels from the beginning of the day and reduce the urge for sugary foods later on.

Snacking can also be our downfall when we're tired and busy looking after a newborn. Explore healthier snacking options as you go through pregnancy; try replacing chocolate with nuts, start shifting to dark chocolate over milk chocolate, and try chia seed puddings, kefir, and berries. The options are endless. Enjoy discovering and trying healthier snacking options now so that as you transition into motherhood, you can prepare them on autopilot and don't risk reaching for the muffins and crisps.

FRESHEN UP

This might seem so obvious, but studies have found that 40 percent of adults are confused about how much they should be drinking, and over 40 percent of adults do not think they are drinking enough throughout the day.[xiv] Staying hydrated is crucial for your overall wellbeing, especially during and after pregnancy. Physically, proper hydration supports essential bodily functions, including regulating body temperature and aiding digestion. It also helps keep your skin healthy and can improve joint and muscle function, reducing the likelihood of cramps and fatigue.

For the mind, hydration is crucial for cognitive function. Staying hydrated can enhance concentration, memory, and overall mental clarity whilst also reducing feelings of fatigue and irritability.

On the other hand, not drinking enough can lead to dehydration, which can bring on headaches, mood swings, and a decrease in mental performance. Ensuring you're well-hydrated supports your physical wellbeing and mental sharpness, fostering a balanced and energised state throughout the day.

Things to Try:

Pregnant women are generally advised to drink about eight to twelve cups (two to three litres) of water daily to meet their hydration needs. Find a water bottle that will work for you—a trendy one, a sporty one that tracks how much you're drinking—the options are endless. Then, always keep the bottle with you, as it can serve as a constant reminder to drink water throughout the day. Coconut water, natural electrolyte drinks (without artificial colourings or additives), or even homemade solutions (like water with a pinch of salt and a squeeze of lemon) can be good options if plain old water isn't your thing. Enjoy discovering new recipes to infuse your water with fruits or veg to add taste and nutrients. As always, it's best to consult your healthcare provider before adding new supplements or drinks to your diet during pregnancy to ensure they align with your health needs.

DID YOU KNOW?

Mindful eating involves paying full attention to the eating experience, including your food's taste, texture, and aroma. Slowing down and thoroughly chewing your food can improve digestion and help you recognise when you're full, preventing overeating. Research suggests that eating quickly can lead to consuming more food because it reduces the time your body has to signal fullness to your brain.[xiii] One thing to think about is how you chew your food—yep, we're going to talk about chewing.

Experts have a lot to say about chewing. One common piece of advice is to chew your food an estimated thirty-two times before swallowing—yes, you read that right! It takes fewer chews to break down soft and water-filled food. The goal of chewing is to break down your food so it loses texture. So next time you eat, count how many times you chew and take a moment to savour the flavours and textures of your meal.

JOYFUL movement

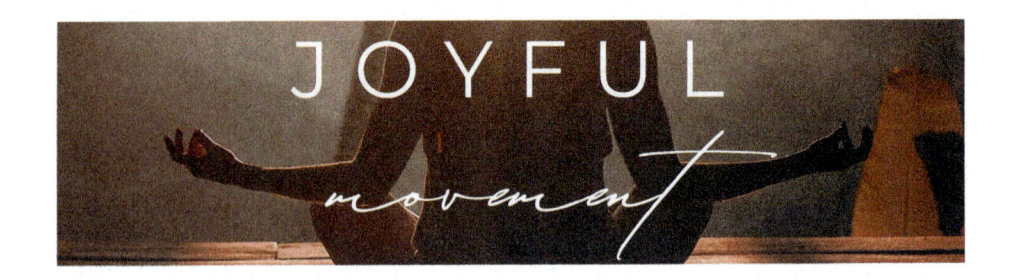

MOVE DAILY

Moving daily is crucial for maintaining both physical and mental wellbeing. Regular physical activity helps strengthen muscles, improve cardiovascular health, and maintain a healthy weight. Beyond these physical benefits, movement plays a vital role in boosting mood, reducing stress, and enhancing overall mental clarity. Exercise releases endorphins, often referred to as feel-good hormones, which can help combat feelings of anxiety and depression.

The key is not in what movement you choose to do, though. The simple act of setting time aside to move daily will ensure that when you're ready to increase the intensity of your movement, you have already instilled in yourself the consistency to commit to it.

For new and expectant mothers, daily movement is especially important. It can aid in managing pregnancy-related discomforts, support a smoother recovery post-birth, and provide a necessary mental break. Even simple activities like walking, stretching, or gentle yoga can significantly impact how you feel throughout the day. Consistent movement not only supports your body's physical demands but also nurtures your mental resilience, helping you stay balanced and energised during the transition into motherhood.

And remember, movement doesn't have to wait until your baby is sleeping; being active with your baby from the start benefits you and sets a positive example of self-care for your child.

Things to Try:

Commit to thirty minutes of movement every day. Whether you focus on your indoor spaces or find inspirational spaces out and about to get your heart rate up, see what works for you.

This could look like daily walks in the park (or on an indoor treadmill) that can continue when the baby arrives or invest in a jogging buggy for postnatal runs. Or think about the things that bring you the most joy: dancing like no one is looking, hiking with friends, or even active video games. You might prefer to consider incorporating stretching, yoga, or Pilates at home, which can continue whilst your baby naps or rests in a bouncer. Explore apps for home exercise or find a gym/dance class or walking group you can join that helps you both stay active and build your local connections, which can continue when the baby arrives.

Choosing to move out in nature has additional benefits as it helps release stress and anxiety and can even give you some vital vitamin D. All you need is two hours a week to get all the benefits! So, make it your priority to carve out this time in nature. It is the best medicine for the soul!

You could also consider adopting the 4-2-1 method—a structured approach to movement that incorporates strength training, cardio, and mobility work in a harmonious blend. This method, often hailed by fitness enthusiasts and experts alike, advocates for four days of strength training, two days of cardio, and one day dedicated solely to mobility exercises. Whatever it is, ensure it increases your heart rate and makes you smile! It is all too easy to rely on the sugary pick-me-ups when our energy levels are low.

REST UP

Getting a full seven to nine hours of sleep may be challenging when your baby is small, but it's important not to stress over it. Instead, focus on finding moments to rest, which can be just as beneficial for re-energising the body. Research shows that even short rest periods can significantly reduce stress, lower blood pressure, and improve mood.[xv] Rest allows your body and mind to recharge, enhancing your ability to manage daily tasks and care for your baby. It can also support your immune system, aid recovery, and improve cognitive function. Whilst sleep is ideal, recognising the value of rest can help you navigate the early stages of motherhood with more energy and resilience. Remember, it's not just about how long you sleep but how well you rest.

Things to Try:

Creating a bedtime routine during pregnancy helps to your signal your body that it's time to rest and sleep. This could include dimming the lights, practicing relaxation techniques such as lighting a lavender candle or engaging in a calming meditation before bed. By aligning with your circadian rhythm and sending these cues, you make transitioning into sleep (or rest) mode easier, ensuring more restful and restorative sleep when possible.

Keep your bedroom cool, quiet, and dark to promote better sleep. Invest in a good mattress and pillows and consider investing in blackout curtains or a white noise machine to block out any disruptive noises or light. The optimal temperature for sleep typically falls between 15 to 19 degrees Celsius – Yikes! After the baby arrives, this established routine will act as a trigger for winding down, although you may need to adjust timings initially.

Training your brain to recognise when it's time to rest will be invaluable as you navigate the transition into motherhood and manage the stress associated with tiredness.

DID YOU KNOW?

Studies show that even a ten-minute walk immediately boosts brain chemistry to increase happiness.

A study by researchers at Stanford University revealed that just ten minutes of walking outside can positively alter brain chemistry.[xvi] The study found that such brief exposure to nature decreases activity in the prefrontal cortex, the part of the brain involved in rumination or repetitive negative thinking. This shift in brain activity reduces stress and anxiety levels whilst improving mood and cognitive function. **The findings emphasise the profound impact a short walk in nature can have on mental health, promoting a simple yet effective way to enhance overall wellbeing.**

Inspiring Your Body
Toolkit

Reflect on all the different things you can try - which ones could work for you to incorporate into your daily/weekly life? One or two will be plenty. Take the wellbeing toolkit template and continue to fill it out. Remember, try these out for three weeks; if they just aren't working, then come back and revisit some of the other exercises to see if something else might work better for you. Remain curious; nothing is set in stone. Learn what resonates with you over time and tweak your toolkit to fit your lifestyle and your values.

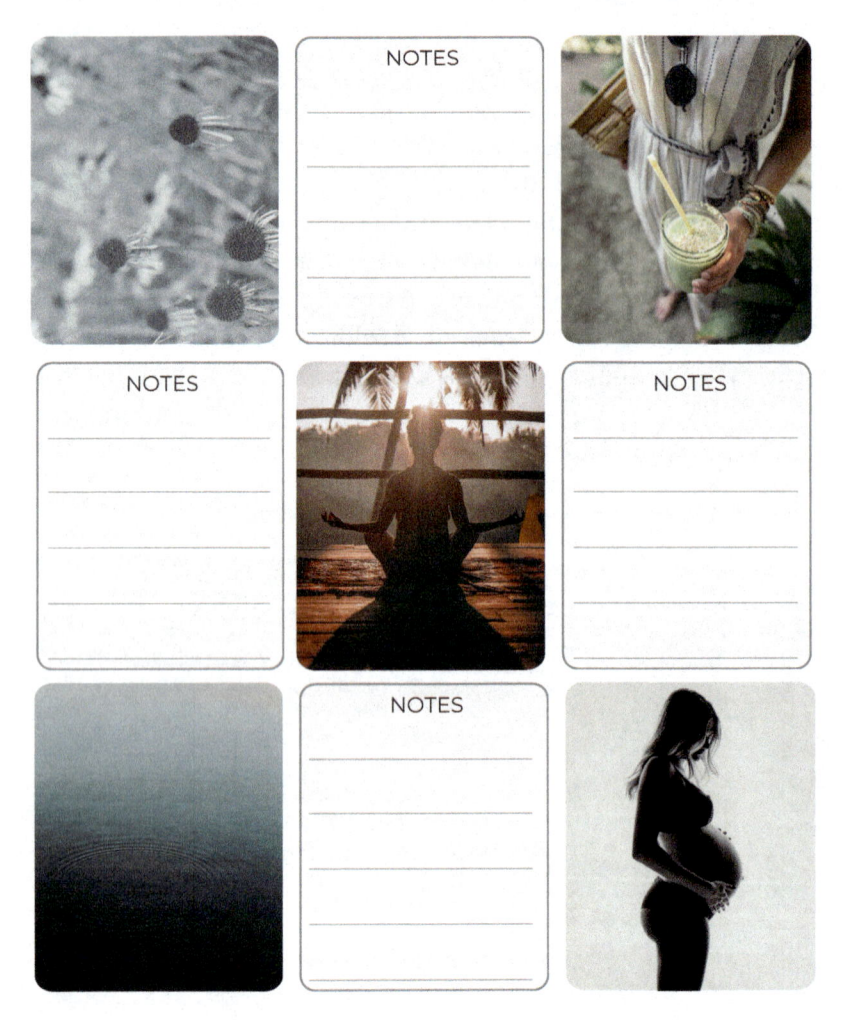

NOTES

NOTES

NOTES

NOTES

A Quick Recap

The female body's ability to bring new life into the world is extraordinary, and understanding the changes and needs during the postpartum period is essential for a smooth transition into motherhood. Focusing on what you eat and how to move your body for joy will help you to stay strong during these huge changes. They can also support a more natural recovery instead of adding pressure to bounce back.

Key Points:

- **Brain-Gut Connection:** Gut health affects mood and energy; a nutrient-rich diet supports overall wellbeing.
- **Focus on whole foods, e.g. MIND Diet Recommendations:**
    - Green leafy vegetables
    - Nuts and berries
    - Beans and lentils
    - Whole grains and fatty fish
    - Olive oil for cooking
- **Move Daily:** Incorporate regular activity to enhance physical and mental health, from gentle exercises to outdoor walks and anything that brings you joy.
- **Promote Rest:** Resting will become crucial to recharge, not just in the early months but as you embark on this journey of motherhood.

Chapter Six

STAY CONNECTED TO YOUR SOUL

When we focus on the soul as part of our holistic wellbeing journey, we must nurture both the internal and external spaces. The space that once felt entirely yours changes even before your baby arrives. The beautifully decorated nursery is only the start. Soon, your kitchen becomes a playground for tiny utensils, your laundry doubles with bibs and baby clothes, and your living room is filled with activity stations and bouncers. The physical space you once had to yourself quickly diminishes, and we underestimate how much of an impact this can have on how you feel. It's crucial to preserve this space even before it disappears.

But it's not just about physical space; your connections and relationships also undergo a shift. Suddenly, conversations with other women revolve around your newborn rather than mutual interests, and time for yourself becomes increasingly scarce. It's easy to start feeling lost in this new chapter.

Here, we focus on the **Connect** and **Space** wellbeing levers because by being intentional now, you can prepare for the changes ahead, ensuring that as your baby arrives, you remain grounded in who you are and how you want your relationships to grow. Pregnancy is an important time to cultivate and curate not only the physical space around you but also the emotional and spiritual space within.

don't forget to play

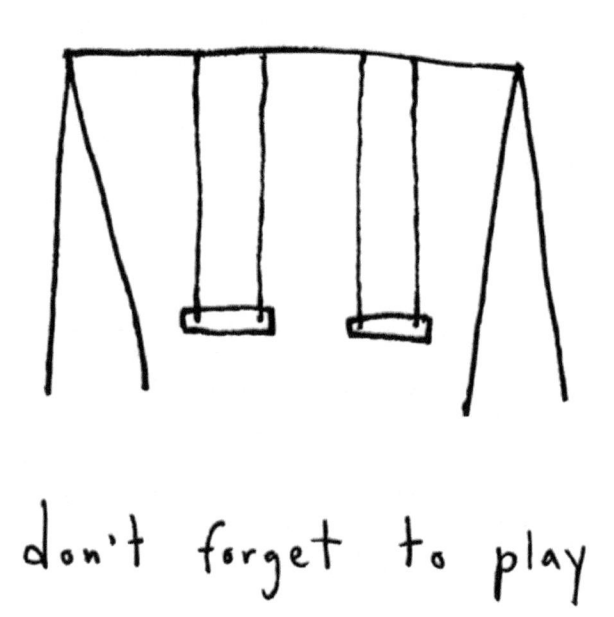

marc johns

RECLAIM
your space

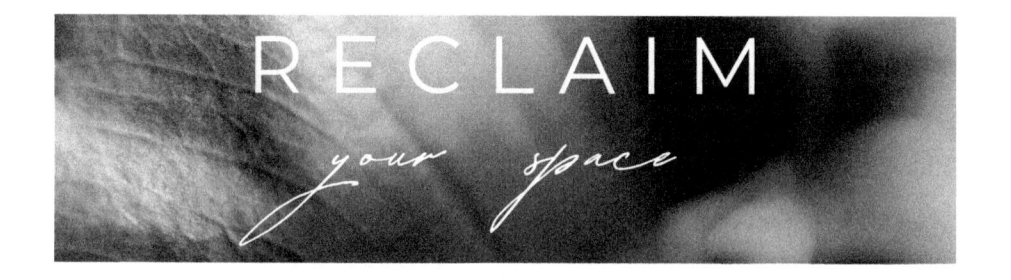

CREATE YOUR OWN NOOK

Stress seeps through your senses, and what surrounds you will affect your mood. So, ensuring that the environment around you makes you feel good is crucial. Decluttering efforts can significantly boost energy levels and uplift mood in living spaces. By clearing out unnecessary items and organising storage spaces, you create a sense of openness and flow that allows positive energy to circulate freely and promotes a sense of accomplishment and control. Feng Shui encourages removing obstacles to energy flow, which can alleviate feelings of stress and heaviness.

As you start clearing the clutter, you should also consider creating your calm space indoors. It took me a while to realise that having my own space to retreat to when times get stressful and difficult to handle really gives me a sense of control and safety. I know I can give myself some time to breathe and engage in something that will help me feel calm and at peace. For me, it's either reading a good book or listening to music with a gorgeous candle lit in the background. Even the act of lighting the candle brings a short sense of relief and calm.

It's time to find the things that help bring calm to your life, too.

Things to Try:

Start by carving out a dedicated space in your home, even if it's just a small corner, where you can retreat and recharge. You might not feel the need for it now, but as the demands of motherhood grow, having this personal sanctuary will become invaluable. Enjoy the process of making this nook uniquely yours. Choose colours you love, perhaps painting a section of the wall to bring a sense of warmth and comfort. Surround yourself with elements that inspire you—books that transport you, music that uplifts you, or artwork that resonates with your soul. This space isn't just about physical comfort; it's about creating a mental and emotional haven where you can reconnect with yourself whenever needed.

Research shows that certain scents can influence mood and behaviour, making them a simple yet effective tool for emotional wellbeing.[xvii] Anchoring through scent association is a powerful way to quickly shift your mood and mindset. By intentionally linking specific scents to desired emotions—such as using lavender for calm, citrus for energy, or rosemary for confidence—you create a mental shortcut that triggers these feelings almost instantly. Over time, your brain associates the scent with the mood, helping you tap into these states when you need them most.

Begin building scent associations during pregnancy that can support you in the postpartum period. If you're looking for energy, incorporate invigorating scents like citrus or peppermint when feeling your best. For moments of calm, lavender is a timeless choice known for its soothing properties. Need a boost of confidence? Reach for scents like sandalwood or jasmine, which can elevate your mood.

NATURE IS YOUR BEST FRIEND

Nature profoundly impacts our wellbeing, offering both physical and mental benefits. Bring the outdoors inside by incorporating safe, beautiful plants into your home or using nature-inspired wallpapers and artwork to create a calming environment. Additionally, make it a habit to get outside as soon as possible in the mornings. Exposure to natural light early in the day helps set your circadian rhythms, regulating your sleep patterns and boosting your mood. This practice will not only benefit you during pregnancy but will also help your baby establish healthy rhythms. Embracing the natural world, both indoors and out, can be a powerful way to reclaim your space and nourish your soul as you prepare for motherhood.

Things to Try:

Build a daily routine that flows with your circadian rhythm. Think about what you see the moment you wake up. How do you get exposure to sunlight early on? Where are the spaces outdoors that bring you peace and calm? How do you use your lighting to reflect nature's cycle and encourage sleep towards the end of the day?

Getting early morning sunlight and connecting with nature offers numerous benefits. Morning sunlight helps set your circadian rhythm by signalling to your brain that it's time to wake up, regulating your sleep-wake cycle, boosting mood, and enhancing alertness. Additionally, spending time in nature reduces stress, improves mental health, and fosters mindfulness, helping you feel more grounded and connected to yourself. Aim for at least fifteen to thirty minutes of sunlight within the first hour of waking to improve sleep quality, overall wellbeing, creativity, focus, and happiness.

BUILD your connections

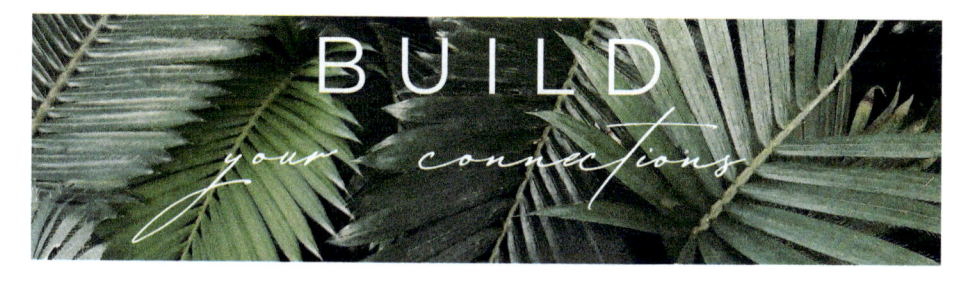

PARTNERSHIP OVER PARENTING

One of the most important connections you'll need to nurture is with your partner or key family members who will be closely involved in raising your child. It's essential to align your parenting styles and expectations before your baby arrives. Open conversations are critical—discuss how you envision your roles, how you'll handle disagreements, and what support you'll need from each other.

Things to Try:

Consider setting aside time for regular check-ins with your partner, perhaps over a weekly date night or simple and quick daily check-ins where you can openly discuss any concerns or adjustments. Engage in activities like attending parenting classes together, reading the same parenting books, or even creating a shared vision board for your family life. These shared experiences can strengthen your partnership and ensure you're both on the same page as you embark on this new journey.

CONNECT TO YOURSELF

Amidst the whirlwind of pregnancy and motherhood, losing sight of your identity is common. Staying connected to your sense of self is vital for maintaining balance and wellbeing. In the Motherhood Mindset Shifts chapter, there are lots of practical things you can do to build up a strong sense of self during pregnancy that can put you in good stead as you transition into motherhood.

Let's also think back to the importance of joy. This is your moment to connect back to yourself and energise yourself.

Things to Try:

Try to ring-fence one hour every week, which is solely yours—I call this the **Happy Hour** - an hour where you can disconnect from responsibilities and focus on something that brings you joy.

Get clear about what brings you joy - maybe it's reading, painting, taking a long bath, or volunteering your time to something you're passionate about; make this time non-negotiable. Start building this into your week during pregnancy and arrange for someone to care for the baby during this hour after the baby arrives so you can fully immerse yourself in self-care, ensuring you don't lose touch with who you are. Write down all the things that bring you joy in the list below and use your Happy Hour to focus on any one of them each week.

MY
joy list

e.g. getting my nails done

MEANINGFUL CONNECTIONS

Cultivate Meaningful Connections. Building and maintaining relationships through shared activities can provide emotional support and enrich your life. Engaging in hobbies with others, whether your partner, friends, or community groups, fosters a sense of belonging and connection. This social interaction is crucial for mental health, as it reduces feelings of isolation and loneliness. Studies have shown that strong social connections are linked to lower stress levels, improved mood, and better overall health. Participating in group activities, such as book clubs or team sports, can enhance your social life, provide joy, and create a supportive network during life's transitions.

Things to Try:

Find ways to connect with other mums through hobbies or shared interests, as this can be a refreshing way to maintain a sense of individuality and fulfilment. Whether it's joining a book club, a yoga class, a walking club, or a creative workshop, these connections allow you to engage in conversations and activities that resonate with who you are beyond being a mother. This diverse support network can provide emotional support, inspiration, and a sense of belonging, helping you to navigate motherhood with a broader perspective and a stronger sense of community.

A little word here on your relationship with social media as you transition into motherhood. Whilst engaging on social and community apps can be a positive way to meet new mums and find support during difficult times, numerous studies show that it can also lead to unhealthy comparisons, which can negatively impact self esteem and contribute to feelings of inadequacy or failure. Moreover, excessive social media use has been linked to increased anxiety, depression, and stress among new mothers. The pressure to conform to social media standards and the fear of missing out (FOMO) can exacerbate these issues. Whilst abstaining is not essential, it is crucial for you to use social media mindfully. Think about setting clear boundaries (e.g., think about measuring non screen time as opposed to limiting time spent on your phone), download apps that reward you for being off your phone more than on it, and more than anything, prioritise building connections in the real world.

Inspiring Your Soul
Toolkit

Reflect on all the different things to try. Which ones could work for you to incorporate into your daily/weekly life? One or two will be plenty—take your wellbeing toolkit and continue to fill it in. Remember, try these out for three weeks. If they just aren't working, then come back and revisit some of the other exercises to see if something else might work better for you. Start small and remain curious; nothing is set in stone. Learn what resonates with you over time and tweak your toolkit to fit your lifestyle and your values.

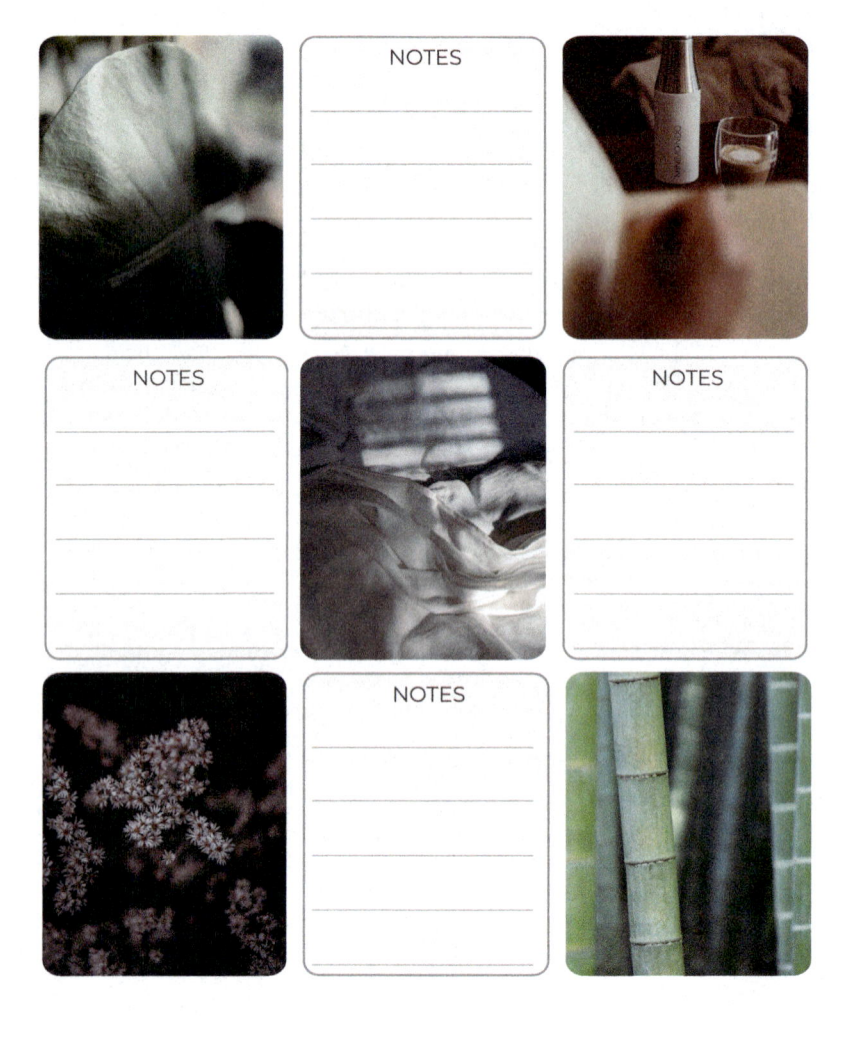

NOTES

NOTES

NOTES

NOTES

A Quick Recap

How you feel is impacted by internal and external factors; focus on reclaiming and nurturing your personal space, building strong connections with loved ones, and embracing nature. Create a serene personal nook, use calming scents, and incorporate nature to uplift your mood and emotional wellbeing. Strengthen your relationships with your partner through open dialogue and shared experiences, and stay connected to your sense of self through regular self-care and journaling. Integrating these practices will foster a deeper connection with yourself and those around you, ensuring a more joyful and balanced transition into motherhood.

Key Points:

- **Reclaim Your Space:** Create a personal nook for relaxation and introspection. Declutter to uplift your mood and use calming scents and nature-inspired elements to enhance your environment and emotional wellbeing.
- **Build Your Connections:** Strengthen relationships with your partner and loved ones through open communication and shared activities. Connect with yourself through journaling and regular self-care and a weekly Happy Hour, and establish a support network to enrich your social life.
- **Mindful Usage of Social Media:** Set up boundaries (e.g., focus on time spent off your phone), download apps that reward you for being off your phone more than on it, and, more than anything, focus on building connections in the real world.
- **Embrace Nature:** Integrate natural elements and sunlight into your daily routine to improve mood, regulate sleep, and connect with your inner self.

Chapter Seven

CRAFTING YOUR UNIQUE WELLBEING TOOLKIT

Setting clear intentions allows for flexibility and fluidity as you transition into motherhood. As you've started identifying the actions that can bring you joy, health, and happiness, this planning can also highlight areas where you might need additional support once the baby arrives. For instance, if you love singing in the choir on Monday nights, ensure someone is available to look after the baby so you can continue this cherished activity. This proactive approach not only helps establish healthy habits but also prepares you for a smoother transition into motherhood.

Together, we will start to put these insights and actions into your unique wellbeing toolkit that you can start to try out, tweak and refine as you journey through pregnancy.

Check in on *your wellbeing*

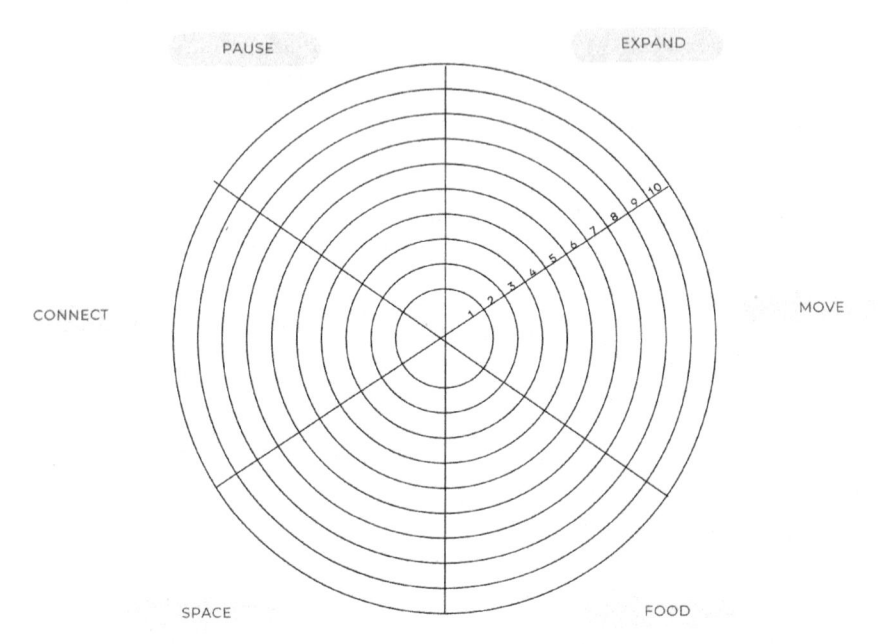

PAUSE   EXPAND

CONNECT   MOVE

SPACE   FOOD

We have provided an in-depth view of each of the levers and lots of inspiration for actions you might want to consider. The truth is you don't need to do them all and neither will you be able to. You must consider which aspects of wellbeing are most crucial for you at this stage of your life across the six levers of wellbeing and which areas feel most aligned with your values and sense of self. **This time, take a different coloured pen and set your intentions within each lever on a scale of 1 to 10 (10 = Could take more aligned action, 1 = Am happy with where I'm at), acknowledging what's already working well for you and what is driving your actions.** Reflect on where you could focus most of your effort to be more aligned with the values you identified earlier. Has anything changed or shifted? This will serve as your guiding star, ensuring your wellbeing journey aligns with your evolving needs during pregnancy and motherhood.

Getting *focused*

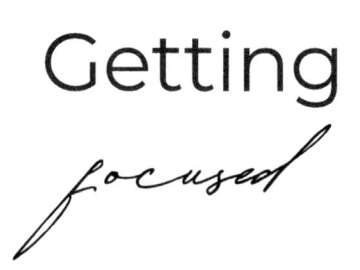

Amidst the changes of motherhood, maintaining healthy habits is crucial. These consistent routines can act as grounding techniques, providing stability and joy even through the shifting tides of motherhood. Healthy habits also give you back a sense of control, which can often feel missing when you become a mother. In this section, we will explore some practical hacks to help you stick to these healthy habits, ensuring they become an integral part of your journey through motherhood.

Looking at your wellbeing toolkits, identify one or two things you could bring more focus to and a couple of things that you're already doing well and want to continue. Prioritise areas that, if improved, would significantly impact your life, your pregnancy journey, and your transition into motherhood. Ensure these actions align with your values and help you thrive on this amazing journey.

Now consider, is there anything in your lifestyle today that you might want to stop completely to make space for your new focus areas? Make a commitment today.

START	STOP	CONTINUE

Sticking to *healthy habits*

Starting a new healthy habit often feels exciting and full of promise, but sticking to it long-term can sometimes be challenging. The key to success lies in aligning your habits with the wellbeing principles we've discussed—keeping them natural, sustainable, simple, and joyful. If a habit feels too big, too overwhelming, or like a chore, it's only a matter of time before it becomes less appealing and we shift to activities that might be more enjoyable but less aligned with our values and vision.

To create habits that truly stick, we need to focus on making them manageable and fulfilling. Remember, every act we take towards our wellbeing is an act of self love, so let's give ourselves the best possible chance for success. For each of the habits you would like to start and continue, work through the following questions:

- **Is this habit truly aligned with my values and vision for wellbeing?**
- **How can I simplify this habit to make it more manageable?**
- **Does this habit feel natural to me, or am I forcing it?**
- **How can I make this habit more joyful and something I look forward to?**
- **Is this habit sustainable in the long term, or do I need to adjust it?**
- **What could possibly stop me from sticking to this action?**
- **What can I do to try to overcome any barriers that might stop me from sticking to this habit?**
- **How can I celebrate small successes along the way to keep myself motivated?**

Your Wellbeing *Toolkit*

Now, take this toolkit and fill it with the practical actions that you've identified that align most with your values and will strengthen your sense of self. Remember, it takes approximately 66 days to make a new habit stick so the simpler, more sustainable, joyful, and natural these are, the more likely they will become a genuine part of your life!

MIND

NOTES	NOTES	NOTES

BODY

NOTES	NOTES	NOTES

SOUL

NOTES	NOTES	NOTES

THE COMMIT- MENT

Today, I embrace the love
I hold for my future self,
The resilient mother in the making.
Guided by a strong commitment
to prioritise my wellbeing
and my love for myself,
I pledge to cultivate
healthy habits,
nurturing strength
and resilience
throughout the journey
of pregnancy and beyond.
With each conscious choice,
I cherish myself,
radiating vitality and joy,
illuminating the path
for my family.
Today, I commit to me.

SIGNED:

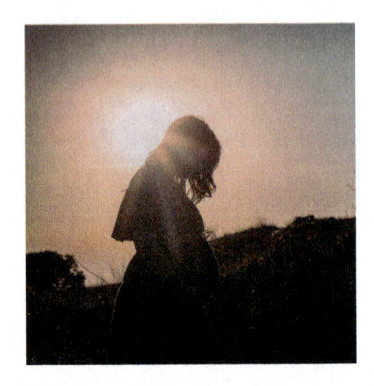

"
A GREAT DAY STARTS THE NIGHT BEFORE.

Arianna Huffington

Staying *accountable*

Forming new habits takes time and commitment, but the key is to stay focused on your "why." Remember, these habits are the ultimate act of self-love, and knowing that will be your superpower in staying on track. To help you stay consistent, we've provided a toolkit tracker—a simple yet powerful tool to map out your new habits across the week. This tracker will help you stay specific and accountable.

When I first started building healthy habits, I printed it out and placed it somewhere I couldn't avoid—next to my bathroom sink. I checked in every morning and night when brushing my teeth, marking my progress with a tick or reflecting on what needed adjustment without judgment, just curiosity. If something wasn't working, I tweaked it until it did. In time, your habits will become second nature, but until then, let the tracker be a fun, supportive way to help you succeed on your wellbeing journey!

Weekly Time Box

CIRCLE MONTH 1 2 3 4 5 6 7 8 9 10 11 12
CIRCLE WEEK 1 2 3 4 5

Monday	Tuesday	Wednesday	Thursday	Friday	Saturday	Sunday
TOP ACTIONS	TOP ACTIONS	TOP ACTIONS	TOP ACTIONS	TOP ACTIONS	TOP ACTIONS	TOP ACTIONS
1	1	1	1	1	1	1
2	2	2	2	2	2	2
3	3	3	3	3	3	3

MINI EDIT PLAN

PREPARATION NOTES

DID YOU KNOW?

Have you heard of the 80 Percent Rule? It's not about strict diets or impossible fitness routines but rather a flexible guide for a healthy lifestyle that empowers you to make better choices in your daily life. It's about stopping when you're 80 percent full, committing to 80 percent consistency in your exercise regime, or striving for nutritional balance 80 percent of the time.

Living according to the 80 Percent Rule means embracing imperfection and authenticity. It's about accepting that life has its ups and downs, that we can't control every aspect of our existence, and that's perfectly okay. By letting go of the need for an unattainable 100%, we allow ourselves to experience the fullness of life, with all its quirks and surprises.

It's sometimes easy to get lost in the sea of wellness advice, self-help books, and trendy diet plans, and we are often bombarded with an array of rules and restrictions on how to live our lives in the healthiest and most fulfilling way. In a world that frequently demands perfection, the 80 Percent Rule invites us to savour the joy in imperfection. It reminds us that life is meant to be lived, not micromanaged.

So, is 80 percent the magic number for a balanced, happier life? While it may not provide all the answers, it offers a more flexible and compassionate way to approach wellbeing and motherhood. It encourages us to live well, enjoy life's pleasures, and accept our humanity. The 80 Percent Rule isn't about being less; it's about being more in touch with ourselves and our genuine desires. Try incorporating the 80 Percent Rule into your life and see how it transforms your overall sense of wellness.

A Quick Recap

This chapter explored the power of intentional action when creating positive changes in your life. By mindfully deciding what habits to stop, you make room for healthier alternatives. Building a toolkit based on simple, natural, sustainable, and joyful actions is essential for long-term success. Tracking your progress is vital for accountability and finding compassion in imperfection is empowering.

Key Points:

- **Act With Intention:** Get focused on replacing old habits with healthier ones that better align to your lifestyle, your needs and values.
- **Define Your Toolkit:** Fill it with actions that are simple, natural, sustainable, and joyful.
- **Track Progress:** Find ways for accountability to start to build habits that become part of your lifestyle.
- **The 80 Percent Rule:** Apply The 80 Percent Rule—aim for progress, not perfection.

Chapter Eight

WELLBEING TOOLKITS FOR EVERY MOOD

We're thrilled to offer you a selection of sample wellbeing toolkits tailored specifically for prenatal women. **These plans are designed to support you through various moods and moments of your motherhood journey, providing practical strategies and nurturing practices to enhance your overall wellbeing.** Whether seeking an energising boost to power through your day or a calming oasis to unwind and relax, we've curated three plans to inspire you. Dive in, explore, and start to curate the perfect plan to nurture your body, mind, and soul as you prepare for the arrival of your little one and the new you.

Calm *wellbeing Toolkit*

FOOD

High fat, high carb diets can change your brain chemistry, potentially leading to anxiety. **Try to reduce caffeine and introduce more fibre, fermented foods and Omega 3s into your diet.** Things to focus on for different meals:

Breakfast: Eggs, Oats, Berries or Bran
Snacks: Kimchi, Almonds, Carrots, Apples & Bananas
Lunch: Salads with pearl barley, Buckwheat, Walnuts & Beans
Dinner: Meals with Sweet Potatoes, Brown Rice, Fish rich in Omega 3s, Artichokes
Desserts: Focus on Plain Yoghurt, Berries & Pears

NOTES

EXPAND

Find a hobby you can enjoy with others, including your partner, every week because **when we feel connected to another person, our bodies respond in ways that help us feel calmer.** Try to find an activity that will bring you joy and that is yours (so that you can continue even after your bundle of joy arrives).

SPACE

Stress seeps through all of your senses and what surrounds you will affect your mood. So it is important to make sure that the environment around you makes you feel good. Create your calm space indoors and find your calm space outdoors to enhance feelings of calm and focus. **Find a space in your home to create a reading nook (or something that will inspire you) that you can escape to whenever you need it.** Maybe even add a lavender candle to your space to infuse even more calm.

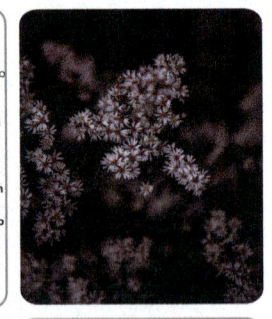

MOVE

Take your walks outdoors: **It's a fact that being in nature helps release stress and anxiety** and can even give you some important vitamin D. All you need is 2 hours a week to get all the benefits! So, make it your priority to carve out this time in nature – It is the best medicine for the soul! Start with as little as 10 minutes and work your way up from there.

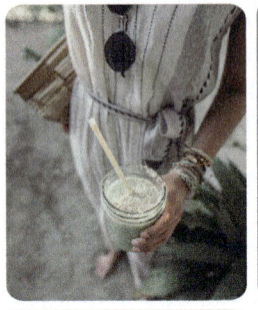

PAUSE

Create a Dopamine Free daily routine allowing you to find an anchor moment in your day and helping you to SLOW down and be more present:

- Set aside 10 mins a day to pause
- Light up your senses with candles, music or a 5 minute meditation
- Take one minute to breath deeply
- Write daily intentions

NOTES

PAUSE

Box Breathing helps to regulate your nervous system, bringing about a state of calm and balance and is an excellent technique to use during stressful moments. Visualise a square as you breathe in four equal parts: inhale, hold, exhale, hold. Start by inhaling deeply through your nose for a count of four. Hold your breath for a count of four. Exhale slowly and completely through your mouth for a count of four. Hold your breath again for a count of four. Repeat this cycle for several rounds, maintaining a steady and controlled rhythm.

NOTES

Energising *wellbeing Toolkit*

FOOD

To boost energy levels and improve mood through diet, focus on consuming nutrient-dense foods while reducing sugar intake. **Excessive sugar can lead to energy crashes and has been linked to depression. Instead, opt for whole grains, lean proteins, and healthy fats which provide sustained energy.** Foods rich in omega-3 fatty acids, like salmon and walnuts, can enhance mood, while leafy greens, nuts, and seeds provide essential vitamins and minerals that support overall brain health. Incorporating fruits like berries and citrus, along with vegetables such as spinach and sweet potatoes, can also help stabilise energy levels and uplift mood.

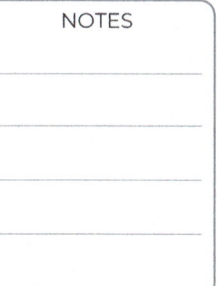

NOTES

_____
_____
_____
_____
_____

EXPAND

Finding a hobby as you transition into motherhood is crucial. It gives you a sense of purpose beyond parenting, providing positive energy and fulfilment. Engaging in activities you love maintains your identity and brings joy amid the demands of raising a child. Sharing hobbies with others fosters connection and combats isolation. Whether it's joining a book club or exploring a creative passion, **hobbies enrich your life, boosting mental well-being during this transformative journey.**

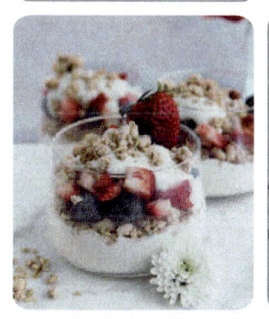

SPACE

Decluttering efforts can significantly boost energy levels and uplift mood in living spaces. By clearing out unnecessary items and organising storage spaces, you create a sense of openness and flow that allows positive energy to circulate freely. Feng Shui encourages removing obstacles to energy flow, which can alleviate feelings of stress and heaviness. Additionally, decluttering with intention and mindfulness promotes a sense of accomplishment and control, leading to a brighter outlook and increased motivation. As clutter diminishes, so does mental fatigue, leaving room for renewed vitality and a heightened sense of well-being.

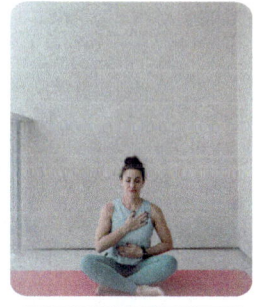

MOVE

Find 30 minutes, 5 times a week, to bring more fun movement into your day. Think about the things that bring you the most joy... dancing like no one is looking, hiking with friends, rock climbing, martial arts, active video games. **Whatever it is, make sure it gets your heart rate up and it makes you smile!** It is all too easy to rely on the sugary pick me ups when our energy levels are low. Whether you focus on your indoor spaces or find inspirational spaces out and about to get your heart rate up, find what works for you.

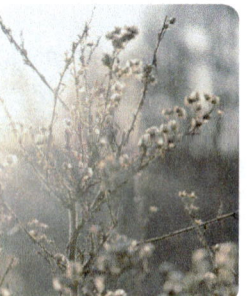

PAUSE

This energising breathing technique clears the lungs and nasal passages, bringing lightness and clarity to the brain's frontal region. Kapalabhati consists of alternating short, powerful exhales and slightly longer, passive inhales. Gently close your eyes, breathe through your nose, and take a couple of deep grounding breaths to calm the mind, focusing on the lower belly. Quickly contract your lower belly, pushing a burst of air out, then release the contraction to suck air in. Start slowly, repeating eight to ten times at a pace of one cycle every second or two. Practice on an empty stomach.

NOTES

_____
_____
_____
_____
_____
_____

CONNECT

Forming connections, especially during significant life transitions like motherhood, can profoundly impact mood and mental well-being. Research published in the journal of paediatrics reveals that new mothers with strong social support during the postpartum period are significantly less likely to experience symptoms of postpartum depression.[xviii] By cultivating meaningful relationships and building a support system, mothers can alleviate feelings of isolation and overwhelm, leading to improved mood and mental health. **The power of connection provides a vital lifeline, promoting resilience and emotional well-being.**

NOTES

_____
_____
_____
_____
_____
_____

MINIMONDO

Clarity *wellbeing Toolkit*

FOOD

Follow the MIND diet - inspired by a Mediterranean diet and designed to promote brain health. Introduce more of the following into your diet:

Green leafy vegetables; Spinach, broccoli
Nuts
Berries
Beans & Lentils
Whole Grains; Oats, Quinoa, Brown rice
Fatty Fish; Salmon
And cook with olive oil

NOTES

EXPAND

Go back to the things you love doing the most…. Singing (find a choir), being outdoors (find a walking/running group), Reading (find a book club) or simply being creative or writing… whatever your passion is, bring it back into your life. This will help you get into a state of flow - a highly beneficial psychological state where you lose track of time and self-consciousness. This state enhances performance and productivity through deep concentration and leads to a sense of fulfilment and happiness. Overall, flow represents an optimal experience where individuals perform at their best while feeling deeply satisfied.

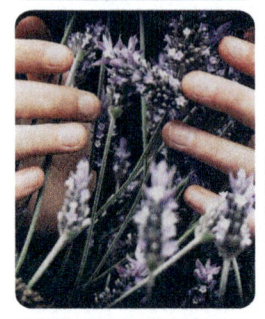

SPACE

Spending time in nature or incorporating elements of nature into your space can significantly enhance mental clarity. Natural environments reduce stress, improve focus, boost memory and creativity, and elevate mood. **To bring nature indoors, introduce houseplants, maximise natural light, and incorporate scents, like eucalyptus and lavender, to further enhance the calming effect.** Additionally, using colours inspired by nature, such as greens and blues, can create a serene environment that promotes mental clarity.

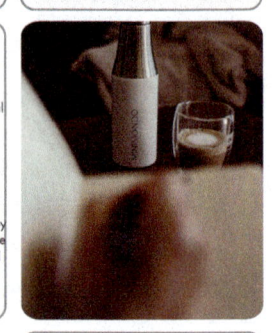

MOVE

Pilates is a remarkable form of exercise that fosters a deep connection to oneself by focusing on core strength, breath control, and mindful movement. **Through its deliberate and controlled movements, Pilates encourages an awareness of the body's alignment and balance, bringing attention to the core and heart centre.** This practice not only strengthens the physical body but also cultivates a sense of inner peace and mental clarity. By integrating breath with motion, Pilates helps practitioners reconnect with their inner selves, promoting a harmonious balance between body, mind, and spirit.

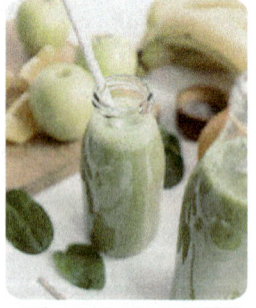

PAUSE

Alternate Nostril Breathing enhances mental clarity by balancing the left and right hemispheres of your brain.
Bring your right hand in front of your face and position your index and middle fingers between your eyebrows. Use your thumb to close your right nostril and inhale deeply through your left nostril. At the peak of your inhalation, close your left nostril with your ring finger, releasing your right nostril. Exhale slowly and completely through your right nostril. Inhale through your right nostril, close it with your thumb, and exhale through your left nostril. Continue this for several rounds, focusing on the rhythm of your breath.

NOTES

CONNECT

Getting early morning sunlight and connecting with nature offers numerous benefits. **Morning sunlight helps set your circadian rhythm by signalling to your brain that it's time to wake up, regulating your sleep-wake cycle, boosting mood, and enhancing alertness.** Additionally, spending time in nature reduces stress, enhances mental health, and fosters mindfulness, helping you feel more grounded and connected to yourself. Aim for at least 15-30 minutes of sunlight within the first hour of waking to improve sleep quality, overall well-being, creativity, focus, and happiness.

NOTES

MINIMONDO 116

> "

EVERY ACTION YOU TAKE IS A VOTE FOR THE TYPE OF PERSON YOU WISH TO BECOME. NO SINGLE INSTANCE WILL TRANSFORM YOUR BELIEFS, BUT AS THE VOTES BUILD UP, SO DOES THE EVIDENCE OF YOUR NEW IDENTITY.

James Clear

NOTES

NOTES

NOTES

REFERENCES

i A survey conducted by Lansinoh. https://lansinoh.com/blogs/

ii The term "matrescence," coined by anthropologist Dana Raphael in the mid-'70s and brought into common use in psychology by clinical psychologist Aurelie Athan, head of the maternal psychology lab at Columbia University

iii AXA Healthcare, 2015

iv O'Hara, M. W., & McCabe, J. E. (2013). Postpartum depression: Current status and future directions. Annual Review of Clinical Psychology, 9, 379-407. https://doi.org/10.1146/annurev-clinpsy-050212-185612

v Dr. Mary Carol Hunter, Lead author, 2019, Frontiers in Psychology https://www.frontiersin.org/journals/psychology/articles/10.3389/fpsyg.2019.00722/full

vi Schwartz, S. H., Cieciuch, J., Vecchione, M., Davidov, E., Fischer, R., Beierlein, C., Ramos, A., Verkasalo, M., Lönnqvist, J. E., Demirutku, K., Dirilen-Gumus, O., & Konty, M. (2012). Refining the theory of basic individual values. Journal of Personality and Social Psychology, 103(4), 663–688.

vii Deci, E. L., & Ryan, R. M. (2000). The "What" and "Why" of Goal Pursuits: Human Needs and the Self-Determination of Behavior. Psychological Inquiry, 11(4), 227–268.

viii Deci, E. L., & Ryan, R. M. (2000). The "What" and "Why" of Goal Pursuits: Human Needs and the Self-Determination of Behavior. Psychological Inquiry, 11(4), 227–268.

ix Envisioning the Future and Self-Regulation, by SE Taylor. https://taylorlab.psych.ucla.edu/wp-content/uploads/sites/5/2014/11/2011_Envisioning-the-Future-and-Self-Regulation.pdf

x O'Reilly, R. C., & Munakata, Y. (2000). Computational Explorations in Cognitive Neuroscience: Understanding the Mind by Simulating the Brain. MIT Press.

xi Mayer, E. A., & Tillisch, K. (2011). The brain-gut axis in abdominal pain syndromes. Gastroenterology, 140(3), 1002-1013. https://doi.org/10.1053/j.gastro.2011.01.019

xii Jakubowicz, D., Barnea, M., Wainstein, J., & Froy, O. (2013). Differential effects of early versus late meal timing on insulin sensitivity and beta-cell function. The Journal of Clinical Endocrinology & Metabolism, 98(12), 5154-5160. https://doi.org/10.1210/jc.2013-2828

xiii Sato, K., & Kurokawa, S. (2003). Eating speed and its effect on appetite and weight control. Appetite, 41(1), 87-93. https://doi.org/10.1016/S0195-6663(03)00035-2

xiv Harris, M., & T. R. Ball. (2015). Public perception of hydration and its effects on health: A survey study. Journal of Nutrition Education and Behavior, 47(2), 120-127. https://doi.org/10.1016/j.jneb.2014.11.002

xv Ginger, L. M., & Smith, L. A. (2012). The impact of short rest breaks on stress, blood pressure, and mood in the workplace. Journal of Occupational Health Psychology, 17(3), 225-236. https://doi.org/10.1037/a0027633

xvi Berman, M. G., Jonides, J., & Kaplan, S. (2008). The cognitive benefits of interacting with nature. Psychological Science, 19(12), 1207-1212. https://doi.org/10.1111/j.1467-9280.2008.02225.x

xvii Moss, M., Cook, J., & Price, L. (2003). Aromas of rosemary and lavender essential oils differentially affect cognition and mood in healthy adults. International Journal of Neuroscience, 113(1), 15-38. https://doi.org/10.1080/00207450390210109

xviii Giallo, R., Wade, C., & Woolhouse, H. (2014). The role of social support in predicting postnatal depression: Evidence from a longitudinal study. The Journal of Pediatrics, 164(5), 1215-1221. https://doi.org/10.1016/j.jpeds.2013.12.039

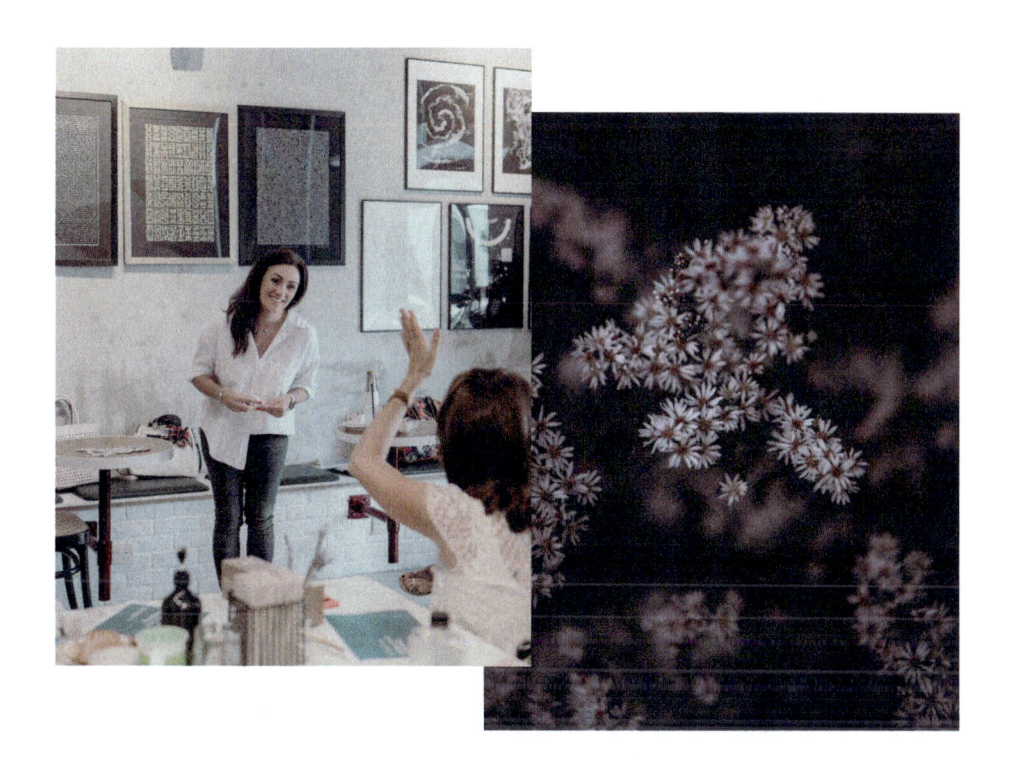

ACKNOWLEDGEMENTS

I am surrounded by the most incredible people who have given me strength and offered me their patience whilst I spent time focusing on writing this book. Thank you to my husband for always believing in me; no matter what crazy idea I bring to him, he always seems to find the encouragement I need to keep me moving forward! And my two beautiful boys, who are wonderful in every way—especially when they bring me homemade churros and ice cream whilst going through my final edit. What can I say—I am blessed.

And to you, dear reader, thank you for trusting me to guide you through this beautiful life-changing journey. I wrote this book for you so you can be ready. And I hope that you will take with you some extra wisdom and positivity on this beautiful journey you're embarking on.

Here's to nurturing wellness through pregnancy and beyond.

ABOUT THE AUTHOR

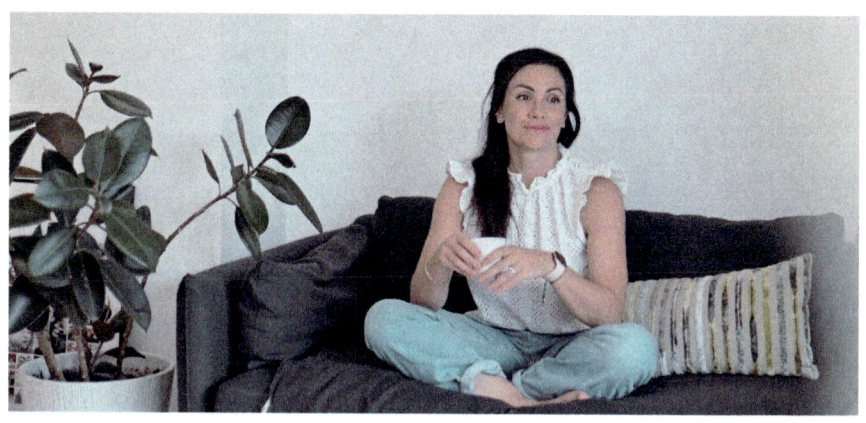

WWW.WEAREMINIMONDO.COM
WEAREMINIMONDO@GMAIL.COM
@WEAREMINIMONDO

Claudia Dumond is the founder of Minimondo, a holistic wellness hub filled with award-winning courses, content, coaching, and products that empower women to thrive on their journey through pregnancy and beyond with a focus on wellbeing.

She set up Minimondo to document her personal journey to wellbeing after becoming a mother, and it soon became a passion. Through her journey, she realised that everything in life is a choice. How you wake up every morning and decide to tackle the day ahead comes down to your mindset and actions. Because of her own journey, Claudia's mission is to support and empower women to thrive on their journey through pregnancy and motherhood. She has always loved motivating others to be their best. She brings with her twenty-plus years' experience as an IIN-qualified Health Coach, Lever 3 Personal Trainer, Pre & Post Natal Exercise Trainer, Gym Instructor, Design Thinking Consultant, and most importantly, mum of two gorgeous boys.

Stepping into motherhood, we embrace the uncertainty with love, adaptability, and curiosity, understanding that each day presents new lessons and blessings; this is the gift of motherhood. The journey of motherhood is both remarkable and testing, pushing us in ways we never anticipated. During pregnancy, we have the chance to delve deeper into ourselves, refining our toolkit for wellbeing and discovering what truly brings us joy. And that's why she wrote this book—to empower other women to be ready—to prepare and not have to figure it all out whilst in the thick of it. Claudia hopes this book helps many women to have a smooth and joyful transition into motherhood.

With love and resilience, may every mother find her strength and happiness in this extraordinary journey of motherhood. Thank You.

Printed in Great Britain
by Amazon